Praise for *Nutrition Authority: Perspectives on Opportunity*

"When we understand our nutritional past, we can take what we learned and apply it to the future of nutrition and dietetics. That is what *Nutrition Authority: Perspectives on Opportunity* explains so cleverly while tapping into today's authorities in nutrition, research, communications, and other areas in the field. This book is an insightful read into the field of nutrition and dietetics and what opportunities lay ahead for new and practicing dietetics professionals. A definite must read!"

TOBY AMIDOR, MS, RD, CDN, FAND
The Wall Street Journal best-selling cookbook author and recipient of the 2018 Academy of Nutrition and Dietetics Media Excellence Award

"I can't imagine a more appropriate or timely dialogue from a foremost authority in nutrition and dietetics. *Nutrition Authority: Perspectives on Opportunity* reflects on our rich history, embraces our current reality, and lays out an inspiring blueprint for the future. These important conversations are a necessary read for every nutrition and dietetic professional's role as a nutrition authority."

CARL BARNES, MS, RDN, LD
Founder, RD2BE and United Nutrition Group

"It is rare to find a relatively short book that captures so much about the past, present and future of the profession of nutrition and dietetics. *Nutrition Authority: Perspectives on Opportunity* uniquely challenges RDNs at any stage in their career to learn from the tremendous work of the RDN colleagues interviewed, to appreciate the nuance of our evidence-based practice, and to be inspired by growing opportunities for RDNs in sustainable food systems and technology. Truly inspiring!"

DEANNE BRANDSTETTER, MBA, RDN, CDN, FAND
Vice-President, Nutrition & Wellness, Compass Group North America

"Knowing your why—your purpose—is critical to your overall success. Reading *Nutrition Authority: Perspectives on Opportunity* underscores the value food and nutrition professionals bring to the communities we serve and provides insights into how we can address future challenges and opportunities that impact global health and well-being. An essential resource for all professionals seeking to understand and leverage vital resources across three pillars—history, science, and new frontiers—creating a true value proposition for growth and sustainability."

SHARON COX, MA, RDN, LDN, FAND
Owner/ Co-Founder, Cox Duncan Network LLC

"Susan Finn is a transformational leader who has influenced many to pursue their dreams in the field of dietetics. She has given back to our profession in countless ways. Her dedication to our profession is displayed in her new book, *Nutrition Authority: Perspectives on Opportunity*. A smart read for aspiring nutrition professionals and new and seasoned RDNs, Dr. Finn's work connects our history and science with where we are heading in the future. As she writes, 'Your success determines the future of the profession and that of the Academy of Nutrition and Dietetics.' We must keep our foundation of science strong and 'The voice of the RDN must be heard.' This book is an inspiring read, guiding us into the future and helping us find our voices."

JASON ROBERTS, RDN, LD, CDCES, FAND
Past president, Ohio Academy of Nutrition and Dietetics

"Students and dietitians will be captivated and proud of their profession reading Susan Finn's *Nutrition Authority: Perspectives on Opportunity* that captures the inspiration of being a dietitian, the profession's contribution to contemporary history, groundbreaking science, and a future that is unlimited. Susan brings the joy of dietetics alive."

KAY N. WOLF, PHD, RDN, LD, FAND
The Ohio State University

NUTRITION AUTHORITY

Perspectives on Opportunity

Susan Finn, PhD, RDN, FAND

with Jane Grant Tougas

eat right. Academy of Nutrition and Dietetics

.eat right. Academy of Nutrition and Dietetics

Academy of Nutrition and Dietetics
120 S. Riverside Plaza, Suite 2190
Chicago, IL 60606

Nutrition Authority: Perspectives on Opportunity

ISBN 978-0-88091-223-5 (print)
ISBN 978-0-88091-224-2 (eBook)
Catalog Number 223522 (print)
Catalog Number 223522e (eBook)

10   9   8   7   6   5   4   3   2   1

For more information on the Academy of Nutrition and Dietetics, visit the Academy of Nutrition and Dietetics website (www.eatright.org).

Names: Finn, Susan Calvert, author. | Tougas, Jane Grant, author.
Title: Nutrition authority : perspectives on opportunity / Susan Finn, PhD,
    RDN, FAND with Jane Grant Tougas.
Description: Chicago : Academy of Nutrition and Dietetics, 2022. | Includes
    bibliographical references.
Identifiers: LCCN 2022016553 (print) | LCCN 2022016554 (ebook) | ISBN
    9780880912235 (hardcover) | ISBN 9780880912242 (ebook)
Subjects: LCSH: Nutrition. | Nutritionists--History. | Dietitians--History.
Classification: LCC RA784 .F539 2022 (print) | LCC RA784 (ebook) | DDC
    613.2--dc23/eng/20220503
LC record available at https://lccn.loc.gov/2022016553
LC ebook record available at https://lccn.loc.gov/2022016554

Contents

ABOUT THE AUTHOR vi

FOREWORD.. ix

PREFACE xi

ACKNOWLEDGMENTS xiv

Introduction 1

History... 4

Science 5

New Frontiers 6

Section One: *Discovery Through the Lens of History* 9

Changemakers 13

The Value of History 24

The Impact of World Wars 27

    World War I.. 27

    Post–World War I.. 33

World War II.. 34

Post–World War II.. 38

Legacy of Social Change 39

The Progressive Era 39

Feminism.. 41

The Great Society... 45

Medicare and Medicaid... 46

Senate Select Committee on Nutrition and Human Needs......... 48

Consequences of Economic Revolution 52

Section Two: *Science: The Foundation of*
Our Profession **59**

Understanding Evidence 63

Research Under Scrutiny 74

Improving Nutrition Research....................................... 76

Crafting and Delivering Messages With Authority 81

Section Three: *New Frontiers: Applying Research to*
Achieve Our Vision **91**

The Food System 96

Information Technology 112

Telehealth 115

What Makes Data "Big"?.. 116

Artificial Intelligence.. 120

Personalized Nutrition 121

Research: The Foundation for the Future 127

Epilogue.. 135

Knowledge, Communication, and Collaboration:
Essential Elements 136

History, Science, and New Frontiers:
My Hopes for the Profession 137

CONTINUING PROFESSIONAL EDUCATION............................. 140

III

About the Author

Susan Finn, PhD, RDN, FAND is a recognized leader and a respected communicator in food, nutrition, and health. As a top-level advisor to professional societies, educational institutions, governmental bodies, and industry professionals, Dr Finn evaluates, interprets, and brings context to nutrition research and its implications.

After graduating with a bachelor of science degree in education from Bowling Green State University, Dr Finn went on to earn a master of science degree in public health nutrition at Case Western Reserve University and a PhD in nutrition science from The Ohio State University. Both Ohio State and Bowling Green have honored her with distinguished alumni awards.

For nearly 30 years, Dr Finn headed nutrition services for the Ross Products Division of Abbott Laboratories (now Abbott Nutrition), where she advocated for making nutrition screening and support integral elements of health care. She was the chief architect behind multifaceted campaigns to advance nutrition support, particularly for women, the elderly, and those with diseases placing them at nutritional risk.

Dr Finn has served as president of the Academy of Nutrition and Dietetics, the largest organization of nutrition and dietetics practitioners in the world, which supports more than 100,000 credential practitioners. She has also served as chair of the Academy of Nutrition and Dietetics Foundation. Dr Finn remains deeply involved in championing dietetics professionals as nutrition authorities. She has received the Academy of Nutrition and Dietetics Medallion Award, presented the Academy of Nutrition and Dietetics prestigious Distinguished Lecture Award (formerly the Lenna Frances Cooper Memorial Lecture Award), and has received the Lifetime Achievement Award (formerly the Marjorie Hulsizer Copher Award), the highest honor bestowed by the Academy of Nutrition and Dietetics. As cochair of the Academy of Nutrition and Dietetics Second Century Initiative, she has been intimately involved in shaping the organization's future direction. Over the past several years, Dr Finn has focused on strengthening the authority of registered dietitians as the profession moves into its second century, effectively communicating food and nutrition science, and exploring the intersection of food, nutrition, agriculture, and sustainability.

Dr Finn serves on the board of the Royal Academy of Science International Trust and participated in the inaugural World Women's Health and Development Forum at the United Nations. As a result of this initiative, the United Nations General Assembly adopted a groundbreaking resolution to establish an annual International Day of Women and Girls in Science.

Dr Finn has been honored for her leadership in health and nutrition. President George W. Bush appointed Dr Finn to the President's Council on Physical Fitness and Sports. In 2014, then Speaker of the House John Boehner appointed Dr Finn to the National Commission on Hunger, which assessed the hunger crisis in this country and recommended how government along with private and public partners could respond.

Dr Finn is widely published in professional journals and consumer magazines. She is coauthor of two books: *The Real Life Nutrition Book: Making the Right Food Choices Without Changing Your Lifestyle* published by Penguin Books and *The American Dietetic Association Guide to Women's Nutrition for Healthy Living* published by Perigee.

Foreword

I HAD THE GOOD FORTUNE OF MEETING SUSAN FINN WHILE we were both pursuing our PhD degrees at The Ohio State University. As Dr Finn was completing her PhD in 1972, I was beginning to work on mine.

I have followed her amazing career for several decades. Without question, Dr Finn has been a trailblazer, making significant contributions to policy, corporate nutrition, higher education, and the nonprofit sector. She is highly respected as a leading nutrition authority and strategist. In recognition of her many accomplishments, the Academy of Nutrition and Dietetics has honored her with the prestigious Marjorie Hulsizer Copher Award, the highest honor they bestow. Similarly, both The Ohio State University and Bowling Green University have recognized her as an outstanding graduate.

I can say with complete confidence that Dr Finn's book *Nutrition Authority: Perspectives on Opportunity* should be required reading for all students who aspire to a career in food, nutrition, and dietetics.

In the first section, Dr Finn focuses on one of her favorite topics: history. She emphasizes that understanding the past is key to navigating the future and demonstrates the concept by highlighting significant historical events that laid the foundation for the food, nutrition, and dietetics profession.

Dr Finn then turns her attention to the importance of understanding nutrition science in the second section. Asking the right questions and vigorously pursuing meaningful answers are the building blocks of our profession, and they are essential to being a credible and influential authority.

In the third section, Dr Finn explores the complexity of food systems. Understanding the elements of global food systems and their synergy empowers food, nutrition, and dietetics professionals to think comprehensively about their contributions to health along a broad spectrum of opportunities. In addition, as the profession entered its second century in 2017, using technology to expertly deploy information is fundamental to assuming our rightful place as an authoritative voice and to communicating effectively with colleagues and consumers.

I hope you find *Nutrition Authority: Perspectives on Opportunity* an inspiring read and an incentive to move the food, nutrition, and dietetics profession forward.

Judy Bonner, RDN, PhD
28th President of the University of Alabama
50-Year Member of the Academy of
Nutrition and Dietetics

III

Preface

WHY DID I WRITE THIS BOOK? THIS IS AN EASY QUESTION for me to answer: I wrote *Nutrition Authority: Perspectives on Opportunity* as an expression of my dedication and commitment to the profession of food, nutrition, and dietetics. I hope my words motivate nutrition and dietetics students, registered dietitians, and dietetic technicians newly entering the profession, and seasoned professionals to take on challenges and new opportunities that reflect our authority on these fronts.

My appreciation for our profession runs deep. My registered dietitian nutritionist (RDN) friends and colleagues have always been a source of strength and inspiration for me. The principles and values of the profession encourage me to do good work and strive for the best. My work with the Academy of Nutrition and Dietetics has given me leadership opportunities that remain invaluable in all aspects of my life. I wrote this book because I want to share my perspective on things I've learned along the way. What I say here is not the only possible interpretation; it's simply my point of view. I know that some people will not agree with me.

I have spent most of my career in the corporate setting, even though I didn't start out in that direction. My first job was in public health with Project Head Start, then I moved on to work in education at Whittier College and The Ohio State University. After retiring from a 30-year career at Abbott Nutrition, I led the American Council for Fitness and Nutrition, a nonprofit food industry collaborative to raise awareness about obesity. All these experiences were formative and have helped shape my views about what makes an authority and a leader. I have worked with amazing people who showed me how to turn challenges into opportunities and become a voice that people listen to.

My approach to this book included citing relevant literature from experts and sharing diverse viewpoints to remind us how important it is to understand an issue or challenge, appreciate other people's perspectives, and strive to see the big picture.

As I developed each section of the book—history, science, and new frontiers—I realized how interconnected these areas are and how they have shaped who we are today and will be in the future. I believe we are now witnessing how nutrition science and public health can develop effective strategies to work together to improve health. And I certainly believe our profession can lead these efforts.

I hope this book will encourage you to look at your work from different perspectives and seek challenges that move our profession into new spaces, as some of the new leaders in our field are doing. Fresh opportunities are emerging, and what you do matters to the future of nutrition and dietetics. You are critical to attracting the best and the brightest to our profession and to promoting diversity in Academy of Nutrition and Dietetics membership. All of us have a responsibility to position RDNs and the Academy of Nutrition and Dietetics as leading voices in food, nutrition, and dietetics.

III

Acknowledgments

WRITING A BOOK IS A TASK NO ONE ACCOMPLISHES ALONE. I have many to thank for their assistance on *Nutrition Authority: Perspectives on Opportunity*. First, my gratitude goes out to the dietitians and subject matter experts I interviewed, most of whom I have known over my career. I appreciate their allowing me to tap into their wisdom.

I also want to thank the Academy of Nutrition and Dietetics for its leadership and for providing a wide range of resources for this book. I am grateful for the friendship and counsel of the Academy of Nutrition and Dietetics executive team, especially Pat Babjak, CEO, and Mary Beth Whalen, COO and executive director of the Academy of Nutrition and Dietetics Foundation. Jennifer Herendeen, senior director of clinical content and strategy, and Betsy Hornick, MS, RDN, director of practice publications, provided advice and guidance invaluable to making *Nutrition Authority: Perspectives on Opportunity* relevant to practicing registered dietitian nutritionists.

In addition, I want to thank Deborah McBride, an accomplished editor of scientific manuscripts, a former Academy of

Nutrition and Dietetics publisher, and a friend with whom I have worked closely over the years. I especially want to thank Jane Grant Tougas. (You will notice her name on the title page.) Jane is a talented writer, editor, and strategist. After 30-plus years of working together, she and I are in sync.

Finally, I owe a debt of gratitude to my family. My son, John, a philosopher and historian, brought a critical eye to the manuscript. My husband, Jim, has always been part of my professional life. Over the past several decades, Jim has participated with me in the Academy of Nutrition and Dietetics annual Food & Nutrition Conference & Expo (FNCE), shared my friendships with colleagues, supported Academy of Nutrition and Dietetics programs, and given sage advice on food and nutrition messaging. Jim was instrumental in helping me write this book by sharing his views on content, format, and—most importantly—by encouraging me when I didn't think I would ever finish the work.

Thank you all for your inspiration and support.

Susan Calvert Finn, PhD, RDN, FAND

From the Publisher

The Academy of Nutrition and Dietetics would also like to thank the following reviewers for contributing their time, perspectives, and expertise during the development of this book:

Erin DeSimone, MS, RD, LDN, FAND

Matthew J. Landry, PhD, RDN, LDN

Makeda D. M. Mars, RD, LD

Barbara J. Mayfield, MS, RDN, LD, FAND

Judith Rodriguez, PhD, RDN

I|I

Introduction

S INCE THE EARLY 1900S, FOOD AND NUTRITION PROFESSIONALS*
have contributed to important advances in nutrition intervention, nutrition research, food and nutrition policy, and food safety
standards.

Regardless of specialty and career path, the questions for the
profession—and for you as a practitioner—are the same: How will
we make our mark and shape nutrition care for the future? What
must we do to grow and promote our authority as trusted professionals? And how do we leverage that authority into dynamic
leadership?

Much has been written about authority, and many words are
used to describe it. Merriam-Webster dictionary defines authority as
"the power to influence or command thought, opinion, or behavior." As simple as this definition seems, the concept of authority
is far more complex. In its multifaceted forms, authority is deeply

---

* The terms *food and nutrition professionals*, *registered dietitian nutritionist*, *nutrition professional*, and n*utrition and dietetics professional* are used interchangeably
throughout this book.

bound to trust, belief, and credibility—all of which underpin nutrition authority. These connections must be built over time by each of us as individuals and by the profession as a whole.

Being an authority in food and nutrition means being firmly grounded in science. In a world with instantaneous access to information, scientific expertise is challenged every minute. An explosion of information—only some of which is valid—creates confusion. Today, anyone can use their own interpretations (or misinterpretations) of science to present themselves as a nutrition authority. We see this daily as social media give a highly visible platform to users with differing views on food and nutrition.

Controversial issues (such as the amounts of fat, sugar, and salt to consume) continue to come under intense scrutiny, while newer controversies surrounding plant-based vs meat-based diets, processed vs fresh foods, and sustainability have entered the fray. We have the responsibility and unprecedented opportunity to break through this noise and elevate registered dietitian nutritionists (RDNs) as scientific, rational, trustworthy authorities. Practitioners must listen carefully to the customer, examine the science supporting what is factual and what is not, and provide the best advice, which require a clear focus and a united voice from our profession.

Academics who write about authority distinguish between *formal* authority, which rests on knowledge of facts that are understandable and explainable, and *moral* authority, which depends on the ability to demonstrate credibility and inspire trust.[1] Moral authority is the term used to describe the persuasive aspect of authority. Formal authority can be grabbed, assumed, elected, or appointed; moral authority, however, must be earned through garnering—not demanding—respect.

Formal authority and moral authority can work in tandem. For example, evidence supporting the causes, prevention, and treatment of type 2 diabetes mellitus is well documented, constituting formal authority based on knowledge. Persuading people to manage their diabetes by losing weight, exercising, and not smoking, however, depends on the patient's perception of the practitioner's decision-making autonomy, credibility, and, thus, trustworthiness—in other words, the practitioner's moral authority.

As nutrition science has progressed, the profession's authority—both formal and moral—has grown in significance and impact. Our profession started in hospital kitchens, where dietitians with little or no professional recognition provided food services first for patients in hospitals in the late 1800s and then for troops during World War I.

Today, our profession includes sought-after experts in research, disease treatment, sports nutrition, agribusiness, and more. Klaus Schwab, founder and executive chairman of the World Economic Forum, notes[2]:

From the perspective of human history, there has never been a time of greater promise or potential peril. My concern, however, is that decision-makers are too often caught in traditional, linear (and nondisruptive) thinking or too absorbed by immediate concerns to think strategically about the forces of disruption and innovation shaping our future.

As RDNs, we must think about how to position our jobs in an ever-changing food, health, and wellness environment. To succeed, we must bring a bold vision forward to ensure nutrition professionals are positioned as authoritative voices. Achieving this goal demands our efforts as individuals and as a united profession.

As I wrote this book, I organized my thoughts into three pillars—history, science, and new frontiers—as a useful structure for a broad exploration of our profession. Such exploration provides a more nuanced understanding, which, in turn, enables us to strengthen our position. Throughout the book, you'll find my point of view as well as various other perspectives from respected literature. I also conducted interviews with experts, some of whom work outside the profession and offer valuable points of view and advice from different fields. Most interviews were with dietitians who have made—and continue to make—significant contributions.

HISTORY

I have always valued history, as is attested to by the many history books and commentary in my home. I'm especially intrigued by stories about women who blazed new trails, such as those who secured the right to vote and those, in particular, who established our profession on October 18, 1917, in Cleveland, OH.*

As a profession, our history and our future are both deeply intertwined with the women's rights movement, social justice

---

* Cleveland, OH, happens to be my hometown, and I was born on the anniversary of the founding of the profession!

movements, and the continued need for qualified people from many backgrounds in nutrition and research. Two major efforts will build and strengthen our profession: attracting people from under-represented groups to STEM (science, technology, engineering, and mathematics) professions, including nutrition science, and bringing greater diversity to our ranks. Efforts to increase inclusion, diversity, equity, and access in our profession are central to attracting and retaining inspiring new voices and leaders.[3]

SCIENCE

Science is the foundation for our authority. In the midst of widespread confusion about nutrition, people want to know what *we* believe. It is up to us to communicate sound science effectively by presenting what we currently know, as well as what is up for debate.

One outstanding example of this essential communication is the Academy of Nutrition and Dietetics almost 40-year-old spokespeople program. The volunteer RDNs who comprise this corps provide reliable advice to the media and consumers, balancing the results of seemingly conflicting studies and translating nutrition science into language consumers can easily understand. One pioneer in this program is multi–award-winning broadcast journalist and cookbook author Carolyn O'Neil, MS, RDN, who over several decades went from popular print journalism to producing, writing, and anchoring CNN's news segments On the Menu and Travel Now.

Now more than ever, we need to ramp up our outreach in all areas of dietetics practice and take the lead in analyzing evidence, recognizing bias, reporting conclusions honestly, and suggesting where findings might lead. This is what it means to be a science-based profession.

NEW FRONTIERS

It is impossible to be an authority unless you are willing to look at the future and embrace change—or even create it. Early in my career in the corporate sector, I saw the importance of change and the critical nature of moving forward when the window of opportunity opens. When I was at Abbott Nutrition (then Ross Laboratories), Nobel laureate Maurice Maeterlinck's words were displayed prominently in the president's office: "At every crossroads on the path that leads to the future, tradition has placed 10,000 men to guard the past." This reminder about the role of change, as well as its challenges, is as applicable today as it was at the beginning of my career. While we acknowledge the value of past achievements, we must break through barriers that hold us back from embracing and leading change.

As you read this book, my hope is that you will ask yourself questions such as: What is my role today? How has my role changed over time? What tools will I need to advance my career? What will my future look like as I join other RDNs and professional colleagues to lead the profession in the decades to come?

Where and for whom can I make the greatest difference to ensure parity in our profession and in the care we provide?

My hope is that *Nutrition Authority* will stimulate discussion in classrooms, workplaces, and wherever dietitians have opportunities to reflect on the future.

REFERENCES

1. Seidman D. *How: Why How We Do Anything Means Everything*. Wiley; 2011.
2. Schwab K. *The Fourth Industrial Revolution*. Crown Publishing Group; 2017.
3. Inclusion, Diversity, Equity, and Access (IDEA) Hub. eatrightPRO website. Accessed November 2, 2021. www.eatrightpro.org/practice/practice-resources/diversity-and-inclusion

III

SECTION ONE

Discovery Through the Lens of History

T HE TRADITIONAL APPROACH TO HISTORY IS COMPARTMEN-
talized and linear, which may be the way you experienced the
study of history in school. Some of you might remember memoriz-
ing lists of dates and events. Helen Zoe Veit, PhD, associate professor of history at Michigan State University, specializes in American
history in the nineteenth and twentieth centuries, focusing on the
history of food and nutrition. Her first book, *Modern Food, Moral
Food: Self-Control, Science, and the Rise of Modern American Eating
in the Early Twentieth Century*, was a finalist for the 2014 James
Beard Award for Reference and Scholarship.[1] Veit maintains that
history is far richer than a collection of dates and that studying history opens our minds and allows us to better understand how we
interpret the world around us.

I|I

Interview With Helen Zoe Veit, PhD

Associate Professor of History, Michigan State University

When Helen Zoe Veit began exploring dissertation topics while studying at Yale, she knew she wanted to focus on food in World War I. Putting some parameters around the idea, however, was a challenge. Veit consulted with one of her professors, who recommended looking at the extensive food-aid programs during the war, how people responded to these programs, and what aspects of the programs were carried forward in post-war culture in the United States.

"I was surprised at how interesting the topic was," Veit says. "I was drawn to the cultural story—the food and the people—and to the emergence of nutrition as a respected science." And the rest is history.

By the 1920s, Veit explains, the hard science of nutrition had become a "popular" science as well. "People felt a connection to the subject, and freely issued their own opinions," Veit, a prolific author on food history, explains. At a time when malnutrition and diseases such as pellagra were fairly common, nutritionists had relevant advice. "It was an exciting time," Veit says, "with revolutionary discoveries around every corner."

"This is my idea of history: not a boring timeline of events, but rather a deeper examination of the real people of the time and how they lived," she notes. Veit admits she has seen some pretty boring history in her day and doesn't blame people for thinking history is irrelevant.

But if you like a good story, food history is an especially engaging and fun pursuit. "People in the past were interesting, funny, and flawed," Veit says. "They had to make sense of the world they were living in, just like we do today. What they did mattered, just as what we do matters not just now, but also 100 years from now.

"Studying history gives us a better chance of seeing ourselves and how we interpret things," Veit explains. "It opens our eyes about ourselves, opens our minds, and fosters understanding. It's amazing to see how people's ideas affect what they think about food. A fad diet today may become an acceptable diet tomorrow, and vice versa—think vegetarianism, red meat, and white flour." Viet also notes, "We tend to take the abundance of food we have for granted, but it wasn't always that way."

———

"What we eat," Veit remarks, "is much more than what we like and can afford." There are larger forces at work.

———

In order to better understand the value of looking back, Veit advises dietitians and registered dietitian nutritionists to try to think of themselves as part of a longer history, asking why you have the beliefs you do today and what influences them. The same questions apply to patients and clients. "What we eat," Veit remarks, "is much more than what we like and can afford." There are larger forces at work.

Another way to interpret history is to look at the whole by seeking common themes and processes across multiple disciplines and eras. Scholars call this study of change over time *Big History*. Taking a Big History perspective allows us to identify forces that have shaped, and continue to shape, all professions, including food and nutrition. It is a point of view that helps us understand the past and present, assess and navigate chaotic environments, and recognize the value of cross-disciplinary thinking and action. A Big History mindset reveals cause-and-effect relationships that may otherwise be obscured, and provides a foundation for informed planning and decision making.[2] Adopting this approach helps us see the forces that shaped the dietetics profession as we know it today and believe it could be tomorrow.

The 1917 founding of the American Dietetic Association (now the Academy of Nutrition and Dietetics)—motivated in large part by food and nutritional needs during World War I—set the stage for what would become more than 100 years of growth and accomplishment. From the start, we have carried forward the professional values established by our founders. Today, the passion and spirit of our early leaders is alive, well, and perhaps even stronger as the profession moves into a second century packed with fast-paced change and burgeoning opportunity.

Connecting the dots, discovering patterns, and understanding the interplay of behind-the-scenes forces at work help us leverage history to propel us toward the future. As historian Ken Burns asks, "Why *would* we study the past if not to have exemplars for the present that could guide us into the future?"[3] Our legacy must reflect the emergence of nutrition authority amid increasing complexity on all fronts.

CHANGEMAKERS

Throughout our profession's history, numerous individuals have influenced where we are today and played a role in propelling us toward the future. These changemakers are innovators and visionaries who have examined the patterns around them, identified problems in challenging situations, and figured out ways to solve the problem by organizing efforts and teams, leading collective action, and continually adapting.

Changemakers are commonly recognized for solving social problems but can take action in any environment by tackling problems with a purpose. The following interviews and profiles with contemporary changemakers showcase remarkable contributions to our profession and offer valuable perspectives and advice.

III

Ronni Chernoff, PhD, RDN, FAND, FASPEN

Former Director, Arkansas Geriatric Education Collaborative; Former Associate Director, Geriatric Research, Education & Clinical Center for Education and Evaluation, Central Arkansas Veterans Affairs Health System; Professor of Geriatrics, University of Arkansas for Medical Sciences; President, American Dietetic Association, 1996-1997

"My path to the innovations we made in nutrition support was literally crossing the street," Ronni Chernoff laughs. "Having

worked in a metabolic research unit at New York Hospital–
Cornell Medical Center feeding immunosuppressed trans-
plant patients, I developed skills, identified by one of the
pioneers of clinical nutrition, Maurice Shils, MD, that were
transferable to cancer patients' needs. I applied this knowledge to develop total parenteral nutrition, total parenteral
nutrition solutions, and unique tube feedings for patients in
a sterile environment."

It was that ability to see beyond the checklists and standard protocols that allowed Chernoff to contribute nutrition
knowledge to research being done by PhDs and MDs jointly.
The networks that emerged as she participated in educational programs to share knowledge about nutrition support were essential to her career, and Chernoff urges people
entering the field to use and maintain such networks.

"Dietitians have lost opportunities by not branching out,"
Chernoff states. "Applying our clinical knowledge to identify
what unmet needs can be fulfilled with our unique knowledge and education provides the chance to move in different
directions. The relationships I've developed in the various
leadership roles I've had with the Academy of Nutrition and
Dietetics and Commission on Dietetic Registration, as well as
on the board of my alma mater, Cornell, have provided ongoing intellectual stimulation and satisfaction."

———

*"Dietitians have lost opportunities by
not branching out," Chernoff states.*

———

Chernoff encourages those entering the field to make a

commitment not only to career development but to seeing beyond the horizon to make a difference in the world.

I｜I

Judy Dodd, MS, RDN, LDN, FAND

Assistant Professor, School of Health and Rehabilitation Sciences, University of Pittsburgh; Nutrition Consultant, Giant Eagle, Inc, 1994–2014; President, American Dietetic Association, 1991-1992

In the 1970s, Judy Dodd, then the mother of two young children, was looking for a way to reenter the workforce and reclaim her career as a food and nutrition professional.

"I've always loved food," she recalls. "When the Giant Eagle supermarket put out a call for a part-time nutrition consultant to create nutrition kiosks in selected stores, I enthusiastically answered."

"Whenever I saw an opportunity for a dietitian, I took it," Dodd recalls.

Giant Eagle, Inc was aware of Dodd's reputation through her extensive volunteer work with local health-related organizations, her community outreach, and her ties to the local health department, through which she had participated in US Department of Agriculture–sponsored collaborations with Giant Eagle. At that time, the company operated more than 50 stores in several states; eventually, that number grew to more than 200 stores, with a corps of dietitians under Dodd's leadership.

"Whenever I saw an opportunity for a dietitian, I took it," Dodd recalls. "Being ethical and steadfast in my principles, media friendly, willing to partner with others, ready to pursue new ideas, eager to accept responsibility, and remaining acutely aware of the company's return on investment in nutrition outreach and education were critical to my ability to succeed doing work I loved. And while I was not the first dietitian in the supermarket space, I think it's safe to say I've endured the longest!"

I│I

Ann Gallagher, RDN, LD, CD
President, F.A. Gallagher and Associates, Inc; President, American Dietetic Association, 1999–2000

Not long after establishing her nutrition consulting firm, Ann Gallagher noticed something was amiss—and she set out to make a change. She remembers, "I saw services like speech, occupational, and therapy services being reimbursed by Medicare but not nutrition and dietetics services."

Not long after establishing her nutrition consulting firm, Ann Gallagher noticed something was amiss—and she set out to make a change.

In the late 1980s, as chair of the Academy of Nutrition and Dietetics Consultant Dietitians in Health Care Facilities practice group, Gallagher escalated legislative activities and is credited with having coined the term medical nutrition therapy (MNT). Her hard work and determination resulted in the recognition of outcomes research as a key element in MNT and in nutrition and dietetics being written into federal regulations for long-term care facilities. "I taught myself the regulations for nursing homes and assisted living," she says, "and took it from there."

In the late 1990s, Gallagher served for 2 years as chairman of the American Dietetic Association Health Care Reform team where she helped develop a compelling platform and led a strong grass-roots effort for MNT reimbursement. Due in large part to Gallagher's efforts, the Academy of Nutrition and Dietetics Washington, DC, office and the Health Care Financing Administration enjoy a close and productive relationship.

Gallagher credits perseverance, patience, and positivity as chief ingredients of her success. In her 2001 Copher Award address, she observed, "Dietitians will be more involved in home health care, wellness programs, and retirement communities. There will be less hospital care, and we must remain vigilant to protect and expand the gains we've made regarding reimbursement."

III

Janet Helm, MS, RDN

Executive Vice President, Chief Food and Nutrition Strategist, Weber Shandwick

For more than 20 years, Janet Helm has provided strategic counsel to a variety of food and beverage clients for Weber

Shandwick, a global public relations agency. As a communications professional, Helm was an early adopter of social media who was ahead of the curve when it came to integrating social media into a communications strategy.

"Around 2007, we had an immersive workshop to educate all employees on social media and how it would be a total game changer for public relations," Helm says. "It was so inspiring and eye-opening about how quickly communications was changing." Helm immediately recognized that "dietitians needed to understand the tremendous potential of social media, and jump in."

In 2009, Helm and a colleague conducted a session on social media at the American Dietetics Association Food & Nutrition Conference & Expo (FNCE), where they announced the creation of the Nutrition Blog Network, a unique aggregator of more than 1,000 blogs written by registered dietitian nutritionists (RDNs). "I wanted to help elevate RDNs as trusted sources of nutrition information online, and ultimately enhance their strength and authority as influencers," Helm explains.

―――

Helm immediately recognized that "dietitians needed to understand the tremendous potential of social media, and jump in."

―――

Together with Regan Jones, RDN, ACSM-CPT, Helm created Healthy Aperture, a recipe-discovery site (now retired) curated by RDNs. Helm and Jones are also coauthors of the Academy of Nutrition and Dietetics practice paper on social media.

Helm says her hope is that all RDNs can see the potential of digital technologies. "It no longer simply means creating a recipe-focused blog, which is where many RDNs started. As we've seen, social media is now a major source of news and information for the general public," Helm explains. "These channels allow us to build a business, promote our services, sell books and other materials, and can help advance a point of view to elevate thought leadership on a specific topic."

I I I

Mary Abbott Hess, LHD, MS, RDN, LDN, FAND

President, Hess & Hunt Nutrition Communications, Inc; Principal, Culinary Nutrition Publishing, LLC; President, American Dietetic Association, 1990-1991

In 1995, Mary Abbott Hess, speaking at the Canadian Dietetic Association, was asked what the American Dietetic Association was doing on the food front. "My honest answer was 'Not enough,'" remembers Hess. This was an "aha" moment for her. "We call ourselves food and nutrition experts," Hess notes, "but while almost all dietitians have nutrition expertise, far fewer are truly food experts. My idea was to create a dietary practice group focused on food and culinary education to become the food experts we claim to be."

———

"We call ourselves food and nutrition experts," Hess notes, "but while almost all dietitians have nutrition expertise, far fewer are truly food experts."

———

Thanks to Hess's vision and leadership along with the support of the 164 enthusiastic founding members and 20 corporate founding sponsors Hess rallied, the Food & Culinary Professionals Dietetic Practice Group was founded in 1996. The group's goals were to develop and promote the food expertise of all American Dietetics Association members and create opportunities for new practice roles within the food and wellness industries. Today, the Food & Culinary Professionals Dietetic Practice Group boasts nearly 2,000 members and friends, offers more than 100 hours of continuing education opportunities in most years, and is the impetus behind the Academy of Nutrition and Dietetics expanded food and culture competencies—and it's fun! The Academy of Nutrition and Dietetics *Food & Nutrition Magazine* is a testimony to the popularity of food education.

"My professional goal has always been to translate nutrition into better food choices to improve quality of life and health. This increases respect for the profession and fair compensation for the services we deliver," says Hess. "If you have a contrary view or new idea, become a champion for your cause and develop allies. When you see an issue or problem, look for a direct path to a solution, using time and resources wisely. You will learn a great deal along the way and make valued friends, enriching both your personal and professional life."

I | I

Anita Owen, MA, RDN

Public Health Advocate and Leader; President, American Dietetic Association, 1985-1986

If you look back to the 1960s and 1970s, you will find Anita Owen championing the fight to establish the landmark federal assistance program we now know as the Special Supplemental Nutrition Program for Women, Infants, and Children (WIC). There would be no WIC without Anita Owen.

After earning her master's degree from New York's Columbia University, Owen set off for Arizona, where she worked in public health at the county level and soon became Arizona's first chief nutritionist. But she didn't stop there.

———

There would be no WIC without Anita Owen.

———

When the 1969 White House Conference on Food, Nutrition, and Health revealed a high rate of anemia and malnutrition in Arizona, Owen and her colleagues asked the Centers for Disease Control and Prevention for a grant to improve community nutrition. With $100,000 in hand, they set up a pilot program, which was formally authorized on September 26, 1972, and thus the WIC program was born. In 1975, WIC became a permanent national health and nutrition program, with one-sixth of its funding earmarked for nutrition education. According to US Department of Agriculture data, as of April 2022 total WIC program participation was 6.2 million (www.fns.usda.gov/pd/wic-program).

Owen advises that when approaching any challenge, RDNs must set their sights on a specific goal, know the pertinent data, and identify where the problems are. "Success takes determination, dedication, and good people working with you toward the goal," she says.

I|I

Sarah M. Wilder, PhD, RD

Educator of Dietetic Technicians; Founding Member, National Organization of Blacks in Dietetics and Nutrition (NOBIDAN)

Trailblazer, highly respected educator, and Academy of Nutrition and Dietetics leader Sarah Wilder died in 2021, but she left an enduring legacy for the profession.

After receiving her undergraduate degree from Tuskegee University (one of the prestigious Historically Black Colleges and Universities), Wilder went on to earn a master's degree in public health nutrition from Case Western Reserve University and a PhD in community systems planning and development with a focus on health planning administration from Pennsylvania State University.

Wilder did not let a day go by without creating opportunities for inclusivity, education, and advancement.

Wilder was a founder of the Academy of Nutrition and Dietetics member interest group National Organization of Blacks in Dietetics and Nutrition (NOBIDAN) and served as its executive director for 24 years. Wilder was also an organizer and charter member of the Dietetic Technicians in Practice dietary practice group. Her nutrition professional colleagues, her students, and her mentees agree. Wilder did not let a day go by without creating opportunities for inclusivity, education, and advancement.

From 1994 to 1996, as research chair for the Hunger and Environmental Nutrition Dietetic Practice Group, Wilder helped empower members to be leaders in sustainable and accessible food and water systems. In 1998, Wilder received the American Dietetic Association Medallion Award for her leadership and devotion to serving others in the nutrition community. And from 1998 to 2000, to help ensure leadership in the American Dietetic Association remained strong, Wilder served on the American Dietetic Association Nominating Committee.

In addition to her extensive work in support of the profession, Wilder owned two nutrition consulting companies, developed a 2-year degree program in community nutrition for Barbados Community College, and consulted with the World Health Organization and Caribbean Food and Nutrition Institute in Barbados and Trinidad. A model of determination, imagination, and vision, Wilder set an example of what one dietitian can do.

I | I

Other changemakers are interviewed and profiled throughout the book, including some from outside the field of nutrition and dietetics who have influenced the profession in important ways.

THE VALUE OF HISTORY

In his classic 1998 essay, "Why Study History?" historian Peter N. Stearns notes that knowledge of the past provides a sense of place and continuity, offers lessons to apply to the present and future, and provides perspective for navigating global complexities. "When we study [history] reasonably well, and so acquire some usable habits of mind, as well as some basic data about the forces that affect our own lives, we emerge with relevant skills and an enhanced capacity for informed citizenship, critical thinking, and simple awareness."[4]

History helps create identity and preserve cohesion. "Merely defining the group in the present pales against the possibility of forming an identity based on a rich past," Stearns notes. "Histories that tell a distinctive story are meant to drive home an understanding of national values and a commitment to national loyalty."[4] Likewise, institutions, businesses, communities, and social groups rely on history for similar reasons—to transmit values and build loyalty.

In their article "What Does It Mean to Think Historically?," Thomas Andrews and Flannery Burke assert that the Five *C*'s of historical thinking—change over time, context, causality, contingency, and complexity—are at the heart of questions historians try to answer, the disruption they navigate, the arguments they make, and the debates in which they engage.[5] The Five *C*'s offer a glimpse into how thinking like a historian can give food and nutrition professionals the tools needed to understand the past and navigate the future.

CHANGE OVER TIME Exploring why some aspects of life change over time while others remain the same can reveal not only the impact of major events but also the role of personal history in the big picture. This exploration helps us recognize opportunities in the midst of disruption, often at critical moments, just as the Academy of Nutrition and Dietetics founders did at the outset of World War I. The COVID-19 pandemic taught us about evolving challenges and demonstrated the value of nutritional status in prevention and treatment of the virus.

CONTEXT Perhaps the most engaging aspect of historical thinking, context strengthens understanding with strong narratives and good storytelling. For example, in my long career at Abbott Nutrition, I experienced the importance of context. Understanding the history of Abbott Nutrition—when and how we developed medical nutrition products—was central to the corporate culture. This understanding inspired our employees and created pride in their contribution to improving the health of hospitalized patients worldwide.

CAUSALITY Historians use change and context to form arguments explaining the contributions of multiple factors in shaping past events, to assert the primacy of some causes over others, and to develop persuasive explanations of historical events and processes based on logical interpretations of evidence. As food and nutrition professionals, analyzing and presenting causality in these ways helps us develop effective communication strategies to reinforce the many factors influencing food and dietary patterns and present a sound basis for future research.

CONTINGENCY Every historical outcome is contingent on a number of prior conditions; each of these prior conditions depends, in turn, on still other conditions, and so on. Contingency demonstrates how interconnected the world is and how powerful partnerships can be. Looking at food in a time of crisis deepens appreciation for the food system, from where food is grown and produced to distribution channels to consumers and patients.

COMPLEXITY History is more than one person or event; it is a continuous process. The analytic study of history that tries to make sense of chaos and disruption is far more rigorous and confounding than the "history" that involves simply remembering names and dates. As food and nutrition professionals, exploring complexity helps us see the big picture and create the change needed to succeed in the future. History helps us see complicated issues and devise solutions that can make a difference to people.

Our heritage as a profession is tied to the economic, political, and social tenor of the times. Our story continues to weave its way through the history of medicine, science, and technology as well as through the vagaries of economics, politics, and social movements. Now is the time for registered dietitian nutritionist to ask: Who do we want to be? How will we get there? What difference will we make? A look at the effects of world wars, the legacy of social change—in particular the Progressive Era, the Feminist Movement, and the Great Society, as we will discuss in a bit—and the consequences of the economic revolutions of the past century can give us some clues.

THE IMPACT OF WORLD WARS

Food anthropologist and historian Sidney Mintz tells us, "War is probably the single most powerful instrument of dietary change in human experience."[6] World wars have triggered massive disruption in the food and nutrition arena. These disruptions have not only changed the way people think about food but also have altered the country's eating patterns, prompted new government policies and nutrition standards, encouraged nutrition science, and elevated the status of women.

World War I

During World War I, the rise of industrial food processing, progress in nutrition science, and the development of America's first food aid program changed the way we thought about food, nutrition, and health. Disciplined eating during the war years signaled a commitment to democracy. Being "overweight"—a newly coined word at the time—was no longer a sign of wealth and prosperity but rather a sign of so-called moral weakness. Wartime glorification of disciplined eating far outlived the war itself. The thinner-is-better ideal that became popular in the 1920s owes its continuing dominance in American culture to the notion that morally righteous eaters were, above all, self-disciplined.[7]

"Meatless Mondays." "Local is best." "Eat less wheat." These slogans make headlines today but were just as prevalent more than a century ago. Each slogan, created by the US Food Administration during World War I (1917–1920), was as important to the war effort as Uncle Sam's "I want YOU for the US Army." As young men fought overseas, American housewives managed the grocery list and kept food waste down so soldiers and people in need could be fed. Food-related calls to action during World War I reflected conservation and volunteerism, early nutrition science, consumer messaging, and the growth of food advertising.[8]

THE ADVENT OF HOME ECONOMICS AND DIETETICS

Even before World War I, and according to HEARTH (Home Economics Archive: Research, Tradition, History, housed at Cornell University's Mann Library), "the discipline of home economics (now human ecology, or consumer and family studies) played a vital part in the growth and development of our nation: it strongly influenced the growth of women's professions, and the role of women in the community, public health and nutrition policy."

The field of home economics also provided a launching pad for what would become the American Dietetic Association.

The Morrill Act of 1862 paved the way for land-grant colleges to educate farm wives in home economics as their husbands were being educated in agricultural methods and processes. Cooking schools in cities like Boston and Philadelphia provided instruction for preparing healthy, low-cost meals—initially to professional cooks and later to the general public. In 1884, Sarah Tyson Rorer founded the influential Philadelphia Cooking School and later became the *Ladies Home*

Journal home economics editor and a food editor at *Good Housekeeping*. She was one of the first prominent cooks interested in health issues and worked with doctors to develop special diets for sick and malnourished patients. She is often considered the first American dietitian.

Beginning in 1899, Ellen Swallow Richards, the first woman to graduate from the Massachusetts Institute of Technology (MIT), first female MIT instructor, and founder of the educational organization known as the New England Kitchen, spearheaded a series of annual gatherings that became known as the Lake Placid Conferences. At the first conference, participants agreed on the term "home economics" and coined the word "dietitian" to describe home economists who focused on nutrition and health. At that time, as is the case today, most dietitians worked in hospitals. In 1908, conference participants formed the American Home Economics Association (AHEA). Nine years later, as World War I approached, dietitians established the American Dietetic Association as a separate entity.[9]

Before World War I, relatively few Americans were focused on food production and the supply infrastructure that provided access to food. In Europe, however, the situation was quite different. After 3 years of intense combat, America's European allies were facing starvation. The United States' first response was to become the foremost supplier of food relief, but by the time America entered the war in April 1917, European demand had exhausted US supplies and driven up prices. It became obvious that America would have to conserve food if it were to continue feeding itself, its soldiers, and its allies.[10]

On August 10, 1917, President Woodrow Wilson established the United States Food Administration and appointed future US president Herbert Hoover to lead the organization. As Hoover observed, "The whole great problem of winning the war rests primarily on one thing: the loyalty and sacrifice of the American people in the matter of food." The US Food Administration proved to be one of the most efficient and successful governmental initiatives in American history.[10]

In 1917, Wilson addressed an open letter to Hoover titled "The President's Call to the Women of the Nation," asking American women for help in conserving food and eliminating waste.[11] The following year, the Food Administration published *Food and the War*, which was aimed at college women and distributed to every college and teacher-training school in the country. In it, Hoover referred to women as heroes and cautioned, "The time is coming soon when the souls of men will be tried as never before. They must have the truth that will make them free. They will listen to you if you can give them that truth."[12] In conjunction with that plea for truth, Hoover also asked women "to pursue those studies which deal with food, and to train yourselves for real leadership."[13]

Soon after the United States entered the war, President Wilson also authorized creation of the Committee on Public Information (CPI), which produced press releases, informational pamphlets, buttons and posters, and $19 million worth of free advertising. The core message, "Food will win the war. Waste nothing," encouraged people to eat a multitude of "patriotic foods" that were too difficult to transport overseas (such as fresh fruits and vegetables) and reduce their personal consumption of meat, wheat, fat, and sugar.[14]

These messages reshaped not only how people ate but also the food industry as a whole. New products were developed and marketed as sources of protein, including plant-based proteins in place of meat, a practice that continues today. Local food boards were established to offer guidance, canning demonstrations, and recipes with suitable substitutions for the provisions that had become scarce.[14]

Homemakers wanting to do their part looked for alternatives to their traditional pantry staples. Local markets stocked only a limited number of items and required employees to gather the food on shoppers' lists, tally the purchase, and deliver the items. Self-service grocery stores began to replace local markets. The first such store, Piggly Wiggly, introduced aisles of food open to the customers, wheeled shopping carts, individually price-marked groceries, and checkout lanes. By placing the workload on the customer, these new enterprises were able to offer more diversity of food and lower prices than the traditional corner shops. At the same time, families were urged to become "soldiers of the soil" by planting "victory gardens" in backyards and parks; the campaign resulted in more than five million gardens.[15]

Prior to World War I, dietitians (or "dietists," as they were sometimes called) worked under the umbrella of the Home Economics Association. That changed on October 18, 1917, with the founding of the American Dietetic Association. Disappointed that hospitals were not as involved in food conservation as they should be, Lenna Frances Cooper, chair of a Michigan food conservation program, and Lulu Graves, supervisor of the dietitians at

Lakeside Hospital in Cleveland, issued an invitation for dietitians around the country to meet. The invitation to assemble in Cleveland highlighted the important role World War I played in the meeting. The invitation read[16]:

> *That there should be an opportunity for the dietitians of the country to come together in conference and to meet with the scientific research workers has long been felt. Now that our national crisis requires conservation on every hand, it seems highly important that the feeding of as many people as possible be placed in the hands of women who are trained and especially fitted to feed them in the best possible manner.*

As noted in historical Academy of Nutrition and Dietetics publications, dietitians were concerned with proper feeding of hospitalized soldiers and nutrition for the public in time of war.[17] Many responded to the military's need for dietitians at home and in Europe. Although dietitians had no military status, the American Red Cross (ARC) was charged with identifying individuals qualified in the area of nutrition and dietetics.[17-19]

In addition to serving as civilian employees overseas, dietitians were assigned to hospitals in the United States. ARC records indicate that the number of dietitians in service in early 1918 was 136; by June, the number was 164; and by November 11, 1918, when the armistice ending the war was signed, 356 dietitians were assigned to military hospitals, 84 of them overseas.[19]

When the war ended with the signing of the Treaty of Versailles in 1919, the US Food Administration and Committee on

Public Information disbanded, but the US remained involved in reconstruction in postwar Europe.

Post–World War I

The postwar years brought even more dramatic changes in lifestyle and dietary patterns. Between 1890 and 1921, almost 19 million immigrants—mostly from Italy, Russia, Poland, Greece, the Balkans, Japan, Canada, and Mexico—had arrived in the United States, dramatically changing the face of the nation in many ways but notably in cultural practices, types of food consumed, and dietary patterns. The work week dropped from 60 to 48 hours, giving Americans more leisure time. Automobiles, radios, and movies became immensely popular. Soaring profits and low interest rates made money readily available for investment.[20] Then, on October 24, 1929, the stock market crashed, leaving the nation in the throes of the Great Depression. Once again, economizing on food became a way of life, and the lessons learned during World War I were back on the table.

In the postwar years, food and nutrition research enhanced our understanding of metabolism and essential amino acids. Vitamin C and thiamine (B1) were isolated in 1926, ushering in a half century of US Department of Agriculture (USDA), US Food and Drug Administration, and National Institutes of Health vitamin research focused on diseases caused by the deficiency of a single nutrient.[21]

In the 1920s, the American Dietetic Association achieved two milestones that further defined the food and nutrition profession.

In 1925, the Association developed a code of ethics, further defining nutrition and dietetics as a profession. A year later, the first edition of the then-quarterly *Journal of the American Dietetic Association* was published as a mechanism for reporting advances in nutrition science.

Over the next two decades, the dietitian's role continued to evolve outside traditional clinical care settings into a variety of professional contexts, including social service organizations and institutions, industry, government, academia, childcare programs, and foodservice management in venues such as schools, restaurants, hotels, and health clubs.[16]

World War II

On December 7, 1941, the United States was once again at war. As they had during World War I, food and nutrition professionals again stepped up to serve their country in government agencies and military hospitals at home and overseas.

At the American Dietetic Association's annual meeting in 1941, members focused on their role in national defense and the need to have enough dietitians to meet the military's needs while still fulfilling nonmilitary demand. In response, the American Dietetic Association increased its educational efforts with new training programs and refresher courses along with outreach to states that might require dietitians' assistance in defense planning.

The country's obligations to its troops, allies, and people at home strained the capacity of the nation's agricultural system.

Restrictions on imported foods and limits on transportation because of a shortage of rubber tires exacerbated the problem. On January 30, 1942, President Franklin D. Roosevelt signed the Emergency Price Control Act into law, setting the stage for food rationing, which would significantly affect US food culture and strengthen the role of food and nutrition professionals nationwide.[14]

With the advent of food rationing, all US citizens were issued personal rationing books for meat, fish, dairy, sugar, coffee, and cheese. Dietitians as well as home economists taught the public how to conserve food and make the most of rations. The USDA's Extension Service, created in 1914 in partnership with the states and land-grant universities, focused on educating rural households about agriculture and household efficiency. The Extension Service deployed home economists and dietitians as demonstrators to teach home cooks about efficient food preparation, conservation, and preservation. Once again, home cooks were encouraged to can produce grown in their victory gardens. In fact, the government encouraged women at the time to design their gardens with canning in mind. By 1945, 6,000 community centers offered canning equipment with home demonstrators teaching canning techniques. The USDA estimates that by 1943, the peak year for wartime gardening and canning, approximately 4 billion cans and jars of food were produced.[22]

Men leaving the farm to join the military quickly created a labor shortage in the agricultural sector. During a 1942 visit to England, First Lady Eleanor Roosevelt, serving as assistant director of volunteer service for the Office of Civilian Defense, met with members of the British Women's Land Army and saw the impact of their agricultural work. Roosevelt, known for her advocacy for women, brought the idea back to the United States as a way for American women to make a meaningful contribution to the war effort. In 1943, Congress created the Women's Land Army of America (WLAA) and named home economist Florence L. Hall as its head. The US Women's Bureau reported that the percentage of women employed in agriculture rose from 8% in 1940 to 22.4% in 1945.[22] The USDA Extension Service estimated that between 1943 and 1945, it had placed approximately 1.5 million non–farm women in farm jobs, and that an equal number of women had been recruited directly by farmers or found farm work on their own during the war.[22]

In the final year of the WLAA, women continued to answer their "call to farms," a common slogan on WLAA posters. In Kansas, 10,000 town women helped farm women with cooking, housework, childcare, gardening, and trucking wheat to elevators. In two Oregon counties, 2,800 workers devoted 21,431 "man" days to harvesting more than 2.5 million pounds of fruits and vegetables.[23] Women also worked in defense industries, taking on the jobs of men who had left to fight in the war. The iconic Rosie the Riveter starred in advertising campaigns recruiting women for these jobs.

In addition to its agricultural impact during World War II, the government helped develop some of today's popular convenience foods including instant coffee, packaged cookies, and energy bars. Food scientists and dietitians played a key role in these innovations. In her book *Combat-Ready Kitchen: How the U.S. Military Shapes the Way You Eat*, food writer Anastacia Marx de Salcedo explains, for example, how today's ubiquitous power bar evolved from World War II's Field Ration D (also called the Logan bar), to a fortified meal-replacement chocolate bar. K-rations—individual daily combat food rations—led to the invention of many processed foods. With products designed for portability, convenience, extended shelf life, and mass appeal, the military continues to play an influential role in the food industry's research agenda and the American diet.[24]

On December 22, 1942, Congress authorized limited military status for Army dietitians and physical therapists for the duration of the war and 6 months thereafter. It wasn't until June 1944 that dietitians received full military status with the same rights and privileges of commissioned officers. The following year, nearly 2,000 of the American Dietetic Association's 7,562 members held Army commissions. In 1947, President Harry Truman established the Women's Medical Specialist Corps as part of the Army, thus giving dietitians permanent military status and raising their professional profile.[25] Military careers have created opportunities for many dietitians, as reflected in the ranks of Academy of Nutrition and Dietetics leaders past and present.

Post–World War II

After World War II, with national optimism high, the economy prospered, ushering in an era of rising wages that saw many incomes double in a generation.

Television, radio, and increasingly influential product advertising had a powerful impact on food choices and eating patterns. In 1950, just under 20% of American households had a television; a decade later, that number had grown to 90%.[26] Thus food and nutrition messaging to the public increased via television and other broadcasting.

A look back shows us that although the challenges of the war years created tremendous stress and anxiety in American society, the disruption and change that occurred during this time also created growth opportunities, including for food and nutrition professionals. These opportunities are reflected in conversations with my friend Charnette Norton, MS, RDN, LD, FADA, FAND, FFCSI, a retired colonel in the US Army Reserve who has held various positions in management and clinical practice and credits much of her success to her service in the military. Norton reminds us that many of the issues we face today are deeply rooted in history. Agriculture and the way food is grown and livestock are tended, food conservation and processing, advocating for government programs and policies, and women's health and career opportunities are part of our history and who we are today. The past has helped shape us; our future work must build on this growth and service.

LEGACY OF SOCIAL CHANGE

World Wars I and II were not solitary disrupters; other events and movements also sparked social change and created opportunities and challenges for nutrition professionals. Three of these—the Progressive Era, the Feminist Movement, and the Great Society—were especially important as our profession evolved. Social movements during these eras challenged all aspects of society, providing models that helped shape who food and nutrition professionals are today. Understanding what transpired in the past gives us perspective on our roots and shows us how to navigate ongoing societal change, such as marketplace expansion, scientific discoveries, advances in technology, and global connectivity that create new platforms and devices to help nutrition professionals apply their knowledge.

The Progressive Era

One period of post–world war history is particularly fascinating—the Progressive Era. Although it began before World War I, the Progressive Era spanned the war years and stretched into the 1920s. It was a period of social activism and reform in the United States, and also the period in which the American Dietetic Association was founded. In their book *Myth in American History*, Patrick Gerster and Nicholas Cords observe that "since progressivism was a 'spirit' or an 'enthusiasm' rather than an easily definable force with common goals… [i]t produced a climate for reform which lasted well into the 1920s, if not beyond."[27]

In the Progressive Era, people believed in science, technology, expertise, and education. Political organizations central to American democracy (such as labor unions, trade groups, and professional, civic, and religious associations) were founded during this time. They brought the scientific method to disciplines including history, economics, and political science, as well as to government, industry, finance, education, and the family. Advances also were being made in the science of food and nutrition.

The Progressive Era also saw doctors and lawyers seeking licensing for their professions, such as the American Bar Association in 1878 and the American College of Surgeons in 1913. Amateur "experts" began to give way to authoritative academic researchers who published in the new scholarly journals and presses.

Toward the end of the Progressive Era, the Academy of Nutrition and Dietetics founders formally established the American Dietetic Association. Risk-taking and fortitude were essential during these years, and remain necessary as we advance the profession and secure a seat at the table when global food and nutrition policies are shaped. The collaborative spirit, enthusiasm, and determination exhibited in the Progressive Era are qualities RDNs need to emulate as we move forward today.

Feminism

In 1837, French philosopher Charles Fourier coined the word *féminisme* to refer to advocating women's rights. The first documented use of the term *feminism* in the English language occurred in 1910.[28]

Gender equity has moved along a continuum that is associated with progress in other areas of society as gender equity increases. According to the World Economic Forum, societies with greater gender equity offer more equitable socioeconomic opportunities for women as well as progress in overall poverty reduction, environmental sustainability, consumer choice, innovation, and diverse voices in decision making on a broader set of issues.[29] Highlighting a few aspects of the feminist movement and what we can learn from its history is important as we move toward greater diversity, equity, access, and inclusion in our field.

Historians point to key groundswells of feminism. The first, which occurred in the 1800s and early 1900s, focused on political equity, mainly suffrage—securing women's right to vote. Second-wave feminism, at its height in the 1960s and 1970s, focused on social equity and its tie to political equity. It sought equal access to social systems, namely education, and encouraged women to explore careers outside the home. Second-wave feminism eventually became focused on education, career opportunities, and women's health and reproductive rights. It is sometimes known as the women's liberation movement. The third groundswell of feminism began in the 1990s. Third-wave feminism, sometimes called intersectional feminism, came about in reaction to second-wave feminism, to broaden the scope of inclusivity, both in terms of culture and areas of growth. Feminism today continues to focus on political representation and equity in social spaces and in the workplace, both in terms of pay and access to positions, especially key positions of power and leadership in corporations and government. The feminist movement today supports the elimination of oppression based on societal norms.[30]

Seneca Falls Convention and the Right to Vote

On July 19, 1848, hundreds of women (and men) met at a church in Seneca Falls, New York, for the first Women's Rights Convention, a 2-day meeting led by Elizabeth Cady Stanton and her mentor, Lucretia Mott, to discuss the social, civil, and religious condition and rights of all women, regardless of color. The Seneca Falls Convention marked the beginning of a hard-fought battle for suffrage that lasted 71 years—from 1848 to 1919, when the 19th Amendment was officially added to the US Constitution. If you have an opportunity, I urge you to visit the site of this meeting. My husband and I visited several years ago. What astounds me is how long these dedicated women worked to achieve their goal—71 years to secure the women's right to vote. This is the message they give us: Set your sights on a goal (in our case, the profession's greater good), and never give up. Our commitment reaches beyond our jobs or careers, to the profession itself and the health of the public and patients we serve, and to how food and nutrition professionals can make a difference.

The Women's Liberation Movement

In the 1960s and 1970s, feminists coined the phrase "the personal is political" as a means of highlighting the impact of sexism and patriarchy on every aspect of women's private lives. Prominent feminists made clear that feminism in its second incarnation was about breaking down gender stereotypes and emphasizing that feminism was important to all people.[31]

Third-Wave Feminism

As the second groundswell of feminism gave way to the third, health became a unifying, core issue for feminists, and remains so today. Landmark studies such as the three-phase Nurses' Health Study (launched in 1976) and the 14-year Women's Health Initiative (launched in 1993) brought women and their unique needs into the mainstream of medical research. The emphasis on dietary patterns in these studies brought dietitians into the mainstream of health research. As the late Bernadine Healy, MD, leader of the Women's Health Initiative, noted, "If you don't smoke or drink, nutrition is the single most important thing you can do for your health."[32]

Over the last 50 years, women have moved from having very little voice in health care to becoming the greatest influencers and consumers of health care, empowered to speak out and make their own decisions about their health. Regardless of marital status and whether or not they have children, 94% of women make health care decisions for themselves, and 59% make decisions for others.

Among women who have children under age 18, 94% are the "chief medical officers" who set the family health and wellness agenda.[33,34]

The history of gender equity, especially the suffragists' 71-year struggle, demonstrates and reminds us that accomplishing change often takes many years of continuing effort, too often reestablishing hard-fought gains. In medical nutrition therapy, reimbursement began with diabetes and renal disease. In the future, other conditions will be added as the Academy of Nutrition and Dietetics continues to gather supportive data through initiatives such as its Evidence Analysis Library (EAL),[35] which offers synthesis of the best, most relevant nutritional research on important dietetic practice questions, and the Academy of Nutrition and Dietetics Health Informatics Infrastructure (ANDHII),[36] which tracks nutrition care outcomes to advance evidence-based nutrition practice research.

Like the reformers of the Progressive Era and our own founders, our vision needs to be ambitious, focused, self-reflective, changing, and compelling in voice and action. We must look beyond our own profession to join forces with others whose goals and skill sets are complementary to ours. This persistence and innovative collaboration are what will fuel our future as food and nutrition authorities.

The Great Society

The Great Society, also known as the War on Poverty (1964–1974), is particularly important to our profession because it was during this decade that nutrition rose to the forefront of public health and the national consciousness, and we saw the impact of seminal initiatives arising from the Civil Rights movement that began in the early 1950s. Many dietitians like me built rewarding careers because of changes that occurred during this time period.

In his May 1964 speech at the University of Michigan, President Lyndon B. Johnson laid out his agenda for a "Great Society," launching the largest social reform plan in modern history. President Johnson's plan included an ambitious series of policy initiatives, legislation, and programs intended to end poverty, reduce crime, abolish inequality, and improve the environment. Republican Senator Robert Dole of Kansas worked hand-in-hand with the Democratic president to fund these programs and put them into action. The country was united on initiatives for those in need, and this is when public health nutrition came into its own.[37] Opportunities in government and public health opened up for nutrition and dietetics professionals. As these programs continued to grow, so did their impact on career choices for nutrition professionals.

While the history of the Academy of Nutrition and Dietetics is well documented in *Carry the Flame,* written by Jo Anne Cassell, MS, RD, in 1990, and the updates that followed in the *Journal of the Academy of Nutrition and Dietetics,* as far back as 1970 the American Dietetic Association formally addressed the concern for a diverse membership; at that year's annual meeting, a "talk-in" focused on the need for a diverse membership.[16] Since that time, issues of inclusion, diversity, equity, and access have remained an active priority for the Academy of Nutrition and Dietetics. The Academy of Nutrition and Dietetics website is a good source of additional reading and updates about available resources on this topic (key search terms: practice, resources, diversity, inclusion).

Reflecting on the War on Poverty, I remember that my first job after college in 1967 was in urban Cleveland for the Maternity and Infant Care Project at what is now the MetroHealth Medical Center. This project was a prototype for the program that would become the Special Supplemental Nutrition Program for Women, Infants, and Children (WIC). I learned important life lessons from Mrs Howard, a nutrition aide who worked with the project and lived in the area. She taught me how to communicate with young pregnant women who had very few resources—for example, how to use their food stamps wisely by following a monthly plan. I learned that to help people, you must first understand them, and they must trust you. I learned to seek out people like Mrs Howard who are wise and in tune with the community.

Medicare and Medicaid

In July 1965, Congress enacted Medicare to provide health insurance to people aged 65 and older and Medicaid, a health insurance program for low-income individuals. Nutrition and dietetics professionals did not make inroads into these programs when the legislation was first enacted. Now, however, it is clear that nutrition services for older Americans is a key area in which we could have greater influence. As individuals live longer, chronic illnesses are often managed with medical nutrition therapy and dietitian-provided services. Chronic diseases—including cancer, diabetes, hypertension, stroke, heart disease, respiratory diseases, arthritis, obesity, and oral diseases—can lead to hospitalization, long-term disability, reduced quality of life, and death. In fact, persistent conditions are this nation's leading cause of death and disability.[38]

Today, legislative and reimbursement issues related to the implementation of Medicare and Medicaid have the full attention of the Academy of Nutrition and Dietetics. Working together, the Academy of Nutrition and Dietetics Legislative and Public Policy Committee, the Nutrition and Dietetics Political Action Committee, state affiliates, Dietetic Practice Groups, Member Interest Groups, and thousands of members have garnered coverage for nutrition counseling and medical nutrition therapy as part of diabetes and renal services. To continue to make progress in this arena, the Academy of Nutrition and Dietetics needs data from its members and from research studies that demonstrate the value of medical nutrition therapy on health outcomes. This priority is reflected in the Academy of Nutrition and Dietetics 10-year research agenda.[39]

Senate Select Committee on Nutrition and Human Needs

In the world of nutrition and dietetics, one of the most significant aspects of the Great Society was the Senate Select Committee on Nutrition and Human Needs, also known as the McGovern Committee after its chairman Senator George McGovern (D-SD). A great deal has been written about this period in our history. Reports document the role many disciplines played in the committee's policy recommendations as well as the role the committee played in establishing the foundation for the Dietary Guidelines for Americans, which are the cornerstone of nutrition policy.[40]

The committee, which spanned the terms of Presidents Johnson, Nixon, and Ford, was initially charged with studying the hunger problem and recommending a multifaceted federal response. The committee held hearings during which it heard from academics, nongovernmental organizations, educators, health and nutrition experts, school officials, the medical community, and the public.

Beginning in 1974, Senator McGovern expanded the committee's scope to include national nutrition policy. The committee's focus expanded beyond not eating enough or eating too much. In January 1977, after having held hearings on the national diet, the McGovern committee issued a new set of nutritional guidelines for Americans. These new guidelines sought to combat leading causes of death, such as heart disease, certain cancers, stroke, high blood pressure, obesity, diabetes, and arteriosclerosis. *Dietary Goals for the United States*, also known as the McGovern

Report, suggested that Americans eat more fruits, vegetables, and whole grains and consume fewer high-fat animal-protein products. While many public health officials had maintained this stance for some time, the committee's issuance of the guidelines gave the position a higher public profile.

SURGEON GENERAL'S REPORT ON NUTRITION AND HEALTH

In 1979, the American Society for Clinical Nutrition formed a panel to study the relation between dietary practices and health outcomes. The findings, presented in 1979, were included in the 1988 report, *Healthy People: The Surgeon General's Report on Nutrition and Health*. The report—at the time considered an authoritative source on which to base nutrition policy—presented a comprehensive review of the evidence that links diet to chronic disease, stated the consensus of the Public Health Service on the policy implications of that evidence, and recommended specific dietary changes.[41]

A number of registered dietitians from leading universities, major hospitals, the pharmaceutical industry, the National Institutes of Health, the Centers for Disease Control and Prevention, the Food and Drug Administration, and the Department of Agriculture participated in various aspects of producing this report.

The committee's "eat less" recommendations triggered immediate push back. Some scientists thought the committee's conclusions needed further expert review; others believed that making dietary recommendations fell under the purview of the Food and Nutrition Board of the National Research Council. The committee held further hearings and issued a revised set of guidelines in late 1977, which adjusted some of the advice regarding salt, cholesterol, and animal-protein foods.[42]

The committee's work in increasing the nation's understanding of the link between nutrition and chronic disease led to amendments to the existing National School Lunch Act and the Child Nutrition Act. The McGovern Report became the precursor to the more detailed *Dietary Guidelines for Americans*, which are now issued twice a decade by the US Department of Agriculture (USDA) and the Department of Health and Human Services (HHS).

CHILD NUTRITION

Dietitians played a key role in establishing child nutrition programs and continue to be involved at every level of these programs, from the grassroots to the highest echelons.

In 1946, President Harry S. Truman signed the Richard B. Russell National School Lunch Act into law, thus creating the National School Lunch Program to provide low-cost or free school lunches to qualified students. The majority of the support provided to schools participating in the program comes in the form of a cash reimbursement to schools for each meal served. Schools are also entitled to receive commodity foods and additional commodities when available from surplus agricultural stocks. In 2019, participating schools and institutions served an average of 29.6 million students each day. Most participants are also eligible for food during the summer through the Summer Food Service Program.

On October 11, 1966, President Lyndon B. Johnson signed the Child Nutrition Act of 1966 into law, establishing the School Breakfast Program, a federally assisted meal program that provides low-cost or free breakfasts to children in schools and childcare institutions.

A 1972 amendment to the Child Nutrition Act of 1966, sponsored by Senator Hubert Humphrey (D-MI), established the Special

Supplemental Food Program for Women, Infants, and Children (WIC) as a 2-year pilot program to improve the health of pregnant people, infants, and children in response to growing concern over malnutrition among poverty-stricken parents and young children. In 1974, the first year WIC was permanently authorized, 88,000 people participated. In 2020, the number of people receiving WIC benefits each month reached approximately 6.24 million.

Many dietitians have served on the Dietary Guidelines for Americans committees. Nothing can be more important than determining these guidelines; government programs (including nutrition labeling, as well as hospital and school nutrition programs) and consumer tools depend on them for food and nutrition direction.

Reflecting back to the War on Poverty reminds us that engagement in legislation and policy issues is an essential priority for us—not only in Washington, DC, but also at the local level. It only takes a few minutes to contact our local congressional representatives, and past engagement has created programs and positions that impact the future of the profession and the future of those who follow us. For example, the Academy of Nutrition and Dietetics Political Action Committee (ANDPAC) played a key role in the introduction of the Medical Nutrition Therapy Act of 2020. Thanks to relationships built through ANDPAC, members of Congress are now aware of—and agree on—the need for increased access to medical nutrition therapy for our nation's seniors. This bill is especially important in addressing the health disparities long faced by minority populations due to socioeconomic inequalities and reduced access to health care, healthful foods, and safe places to be active.

As the largest food and nutrition organization in the world, the Academy of Nutrition and Dietetics provides us the opportunity to unite around messages and programs that communicate recommendations and guidelines. By joining forces to engage with others who share our concerns and priorities, we can increase both our presence and our beneficial impact on an increasingly global audience.

CONSEQUENCES OF ECONOMIC REVOLUTION

In addition to the aforementioned historical eras, we also need to acknowledge the importance of the economic revolution of the past century. Like the disruption of world wars and the transformation of social change, the impact of economic revolution has helped shape the profession of nutrition and dietetics. In times of plenty and in times of scarcity, food and nutrition professionals have provided valuable guidance to the public. Whether working in hospitals, public health, government, academia, industry, or private practice, the profession has demonstrated repeatedly that both nutrition science and education on the practical application of nutrition principles are essential to health.

When viewed from a Big History perspective, it is clear how economic disruption continues to change the world and our profession. The Industrial Revolution, in which the world economy changed from being predominantly agrarian to being largely industrial, created major shifts in world economics. Advances took place in the steel, electric, automobile, and aeronautical industries. The advent of computers led to the Digital Revolution—often called the Third Industrial Revolution—bringing with it microchip processing, telecommunication innovations, automation, robotics, and the disruption of massive change at unprecedented speed in almost every industry worldwide.

Nancy E. Roman, CEO of Partnership for a Healthier America, explains that in the post-World War I and World War II economies, "we took advantage of all the new technology that the Industrial Revolution had to offer to develop exactly what consumers asked for, which was very convenient, delicious food that was shelf stable and could be prepared quickly. What we didn't understand or appreciate fully then was the connection that the sodium and added sugar and ultrarefined grains in those products would come to have on our health."[43]

If harnessed appropriately, Roman says, rapid advances in digital technology could offer much-needed solutions to some of the unintentional negative consequences to diets and nutrition resulting from otherwise positive developments during the Industrial Revolution.

Throughout the last century, we have pushed boundaries, overcome barriers, and navigated complexity to combat the food and nutrition consequences of disrupters like world wars, social change, and the economic upheaval of industrialization. We have built an identity and inspired loyalty in our ranks. Facing the future, we need to embrace change and understand that our jobs will be dramatically different in the future. The instant connectivity our colleagues and clients expect requires knowledge of leading-edge diagnostic, monitoring, and communications technologies, and our education and training systems require greater diversity to arm future dietitians with the skills needed in an inclusive global workplace.

History helps us understand what underpins our profession. The ability to think like a historian—to hone our vision for the future by digging deep to uncover patterns and insights, to grasp the interdependence of events unfolding around us, and to nurture an open mind and critical thinking in the face of controversy and challenge—creates in us a mindset that projects the vision, trust, and authority necessary to create a world where all people thrive through the transformative power of food and nutrition.

REFERENCES

1. Veit H. *Modern Food, Moral Food: Self-Control, Science, and the Rise of Modern American Eating in the Early Twentieth Century.* University of North Carolina Press; 2013.
2. Gates B. Big History for everyone. GatesNotes website. Published 2013. Accessed December 15, 2020. www.gatesnotes.com/education/big-history-for-everyone
3. Barnes R. 'To will the past alive': A conversation with Ken Burns. US History Scene website. Accessed December 15, 2020. https://ushistoryscene.com/article/ken-burns
4. Stearns P. Why study history? American Historical Association website. 1998. Accessed December 15, 20. www.historians.org/about-aha-and-membership/aha-history-and-archives/historical-archives/why-study-history-(1998)

5. Andrews T, Burke F. What does it mean to think historically? Perspectives on history. American Historical Association website. 2007. Accessed December 15, 2020. www.historians.org/publications-and-directories/perspectives-on-history /january-2007/what-does-it-mean-to-think-historically

6. Mintz S. *Sweetness and Power.* Penguin Books; 1986.

7. Viet H. The Great War and modern food. UNC Press Blog website. 2015. Accessed December 15, 2020. https://uncpressblog.com/2015/08/03/helen -zoe-veit-the-great-war-and-modern-food

8. McCowan D. How WWI food propaganda forever changed the way Americans eat. The Takeout website. 2017. Accessed December 15, 2020. https://thetakeout.com/how-wwi-food-propaganda-forever-changed-the-way -america-1798259481

9. Home economics and its literature. Cornell University Library website. Accessed October 21, 2021. https://digital.library.cornell.edu/collections /hearth/project

10. Martin C. Save a loaf a week, help win the war: Food conservation and World War I. Remembering World War website. Accessed December 15, 2020. https://rememberingwwi.villanova.edu/food-conservation

11. Capozzola C. *Uncle Sam Wants You.* Oxford University Press; 2008.

12. Hoover H. To the women of the universities and colleges. *United States Food Administration: Food and the War: A Textbook for College Classes.* Houghton Mifflin; 1918.

13. Hoover H. World food situation discussed by Mr. Hoover. *American Food Journal.* 1918;13(11):617.

14. Schumm L. Food rationing in wartime America. History Channel website. Published 2018. Accessed December 15, 2020. www.history.com/news/food -rationing-in-wartime-america

15. Pack C. *The War Garden Victorious.* J.P. Lippincott & Company; 1919.

16. Cassell J. *Carry the Flame: The History of the American Dietetic Association.* American Dietetic Association; 1990.

17. Lee H, McDaniel M. *Army Medical Specialist Corps.* Office of the Surgeon General, Army Medical Specialist Corps, Department of the Army; 1968.

18. Dock L, Pickett S, Noyes C, Clement F, Fox E, Van Meter A. *History of American Red Cross Nursing.* Macmillan Co; 1922.

19. Manchester KE. *History of the Army Dietitian (official record).* Office of the Surgeon General, Department of the Army; 1960.

20. History of the United States, War and Prosperity. US Diplomatic Mission to Germany website. Accessed December 15, 2020. https://usa.usembassy.de /history-ww1.htm

21. Mozaffarian D, Rosenberg I, Uauy R. History of modern nutrition science—implications for current research, dietary guidelines, and food policy. *BMJ.* 2018:k2392. doi:10.1136/bmj.k2392

22. Food rationing and canning in World War II. National Women's History Museum website. 2017. Accessed December 15, 2020. www.womenshistory .org/articles/food-rationing-and-canning-world-war-ii

23. Litoff J, Smith D. To the rescue of the crops: The Women's Land Army during World War II. *Prologue.* 1993;25(4).

24. De Salcedo, AM. *Combat-Ready Kitchen: How the U.S. Military Shapes the Way You Eat.* Penguin Random House; 2015.

25. Hodges, PAM. Perspectives on history: Army dietitians in the European, North African, and Mediterranean theaters of operation in World War II. *J Am Diet Assoc.* 1996;96(6):598-601. doi:10.1016/S0002-8223(96)00164-2

26. 1950s TV and radio. Encyclopedia.com website. Accessed October 21, 2021. www.encyclopedia.com/history/culture-magazines/1950s-tv-and-radio

27. Gerster P, Cords N. *Myth in American History.* Glencoe Press; 1977.

28. Offen, K. On the French origin of the words feminism and feminist. *Feminist Issues.* 1988;8(2):45-51. doi:10.1007/BF02685596

29. Abney D, González A. This is why women must play a greater role in the global economy. World Economic Forum Annual Meeting, January 23-26, 2018. Davos-Klosters, Switzerland. Accessed October 21, 2021. www.weforum.org /agenda/2018/01/this-is-why-women-must-play-a-greater-role-in-the-global -economy

30. Drucker, SA. Betty Friedan: The Three Waves of Feminism. April 27, 2018. Ohio Humanities website. Accessed December 18, 2020. www.ohiohumanities .org/betty-friedan-the-three-waves-of-feminism

31. Munro E. Feminism: A fourth wave? PSA Blog. September 5, 2013. Political Science Association website. Accessed October 21, 2021. www.psa.ac.uk/psa /news/feminism-fourth-wave

32. Healy B. *A New Prescription for Women's Health.* Viking; 1995.

33. Luce CB, Hewlett SA, Kennedy JT, Sherbin L. The power of the purse: Engaging women decision makers for healthy outcomes. Center for Talent Innovation website. 2015. www.talentinnovation.org/publication.cfm ?publication=1470

34. Lounsbery K. Healthcare's primary decision-maker is female. NRC Health website. March 30, 2018. Accessed October 21, 2021. https://nrchealth.com /editorial-healthcares-primary-decision-maker-female

35. Academy of Nutrition and Dietetics Evidence Analysis Library. www.andeal.org

36. Academy of Nutrition and Dietetics Health Informatics Infrastructure (ANDHII). eatrightPRO website. Accessed November 2, 2021. www.eatrightpro.org/research/projects-tools-and-initiatives/andhii

37. Great Society. The History Channel website. August 28, 2018. Accessed December 15, 2020. www.history.com/topics/1960s/great-society

38. *The Power of Prevention: Chronic Disease… the Public Health Challenge of the 21st Century.* National Center for Chronic Disease Prevention and Health Promotion; 2009. Accessed December 15, 2020. www.cdc.gov/chronicdisease /pdf/2009-Power-of-Prevention.pdf

39. Academy of Nutrition and Dietetics. *Academy Research Priorities: an Agenda to Advance Nutrition And Dietetics Knowledge & Practice.* eatrightPRO website. 2020. Accessed December 20, 2020. www.eatrightpro.org/-/media/eatrightpro -files/research/research-priorities-final-report.pdf

40. Table: History of dietary guidance development in the United States and the Dietary Guidelines for Americans—a chronology. Dietary Guidelines for Americans website. Accessed October 21, 2021. www.dietaryguidelines.gov /about-dietary-guidelines/history-dietary-guidelines/summary-dietary -guidance-development

41. McGinnis JM, Nestle M. US Department of Health, Education, and Welfare, Public Health Service. *Healthy People: The Surgeon General's Report on Health Promotion and Disease Prevention.* DHEW (PHS) Publication No. 79-55071, 197.

42. Select Committee on Nutrition and Human Needs, US Senate. *Dietary Goals for the United States.* 2nd ed. US Government Printing Office; 1977. Accessed October 21, 2021. https://thescienceofnutrition.files.wordpress.com/2014/03 /dietary-goals-for-the-united-states.pdf

43. Crawford E. Could the Digital Revolution solve diet-related problems caused by the Industrial Revolution? Foodnavigator-usa.com website; March 21, 2019. Accessed December 25, 2020. www.foodnavigator-usa.com/Article /2019/03/21/Could-the-Digital-Revolution-solve-diet-related-problems -caused-by-the-Industrial-Revolution

SECTION TWO

Science: The Foundation of Our Profession

===========

Science—the art of asking questions and finding new knowledge and perspective—is the foundation of the nutrition and dietetics profession. The science of nutrition is at the core of our authority, credibility, and influence, whether we apply our expertise as individual counselors, educators, translational scientists, bench researchers, or public health regulators, and whether we work in clinical settings, such as hospitals and nursing homes, school food service, industry, agriculture, or any of the other settings in which dietitians make their mark.

Nutrition science exists within the greater world of scientific inquiry. Boundaries between the science of nutrition and many other biological sciences have blurred over the decades. For example, the science of chemistry is now used to study how food ingredients interact with each other, physiology helps us understand how nutrients are assimilated into body tissues, and engineering is involved in creating new fortified foods. The social sciences also influence our work: anthropology explores why we chose to eat certain foods in centuries past, and psychology guides us to determine what attitudes and behaviors influence our dietary patterns today.

Like all science, nutrition science is a process of discovery. And, like all science, it is rife with challenges and seeming contradictions that can make it difficult to provide clear and definitive messages. People want definitive answers, but as the late Charles Krauthammer, MD, noted in a 2014 *Washington Post* editorial, "There is nothing more anti-scientific than the very idea that science is settled, static, and impervious to challenge."[1] Our ability to communicate nutrition science with confidence, competence, and professionalism is essential, and it is key to how other people accept us as an authoritative voice. In the accompanying interview, Roger Clemens, DrPH, CFS, CNS, FIFT, FASN, FACN, FIAFST, provides insight on how to look at research reports to avoid mistrust of scientific messages.

I | I

Roger Clemens, DrPH, CFS, CNS, FIFT, FASN, FACN, FIAFST

Adjunct Professor, Pharmacology and Pharmaceutical Sciences; Assistant Professor, Regulatory and Quality Sciences; University of Southern California School of Pharmacy

His credentials are impeccable: past president of the Institute of Food Technologists (IFT); presiding officer of the International Academy of Food Science and Technology; former scientific advisor for Nestlé USA; developer of graduate global nutrition courses within the USC School of Medicine; honorary member of the Academy of Nutrition and Dietetics. Roger Clemens can provide prodigious advice to dietitians as they create messages for the public. He cautions that these days, when science is often mistrusted, dietitians must be able to distinguish top-line results from the real meaning of published studies. Doing so is critical to earning the trust and authority dietitians deserve as scientifically trained professionals.

———

"Analyzing studies and understanding research are basic to supporting scientific evidence, but earning trust through relating to people as people is fundamental, particularly on the global stage."

———

"It is imperative to identify when data have been manipulated to fit a hypothesis and when messages have been crafted based on faulty studies," cautions Clemens. "The research models have to be based on physiologic rules." He advises that understanding study methodology and quality, phrasing of research questions, study size, application of statistical methods, epidemiologic influences, and other factors give dietitians the grounding to offer science-based counsel to their clients and patients. In addition, interacting with the range of professionals involved in food science as a whole broadens dietitians' scope and their importance in the food system.

"We also need to understand diversity of cultures and traditions as we talk with people about food," Clemens says. "Analyzing studies and understanding research are basic to supporting scientific evidence, but earning trust through relating to people as people is fundamental, particularly on the global stage. The integration of nutrition, food science, toxicology, dietetics, physics, chemistry, etc, are all part of the STEM [science, technology, engineering, and mathematics] curriculum that reinforces the authority that dietitians hold."

I ǁ I

In school we are taught the scientific method, which proceeds through the following ordered steps: (1) develop a research question and a hypothesis, (2) design an experiment to test the hypothesis, (3) perform the experiment and carefully record the results, (4) analyze the results and determine whether the hypothesis is supported by the data, and (5) report the results to allow others to repeat the experiment and confirm the results.

This ideal version of the scientific method—and science itself—is compelling because it is precisely that: an ideal. In real-life nutrition science, people eat all sorts of food in combinations as part of different dietary patterns that make it challenging to attach any outcome to a particular food or nutrient, not to mention all the other variables that affect health, such as exercise, drinking habits, body composition, genetics, and much more. This is just one example of how complicated nutrition research can be. It is little wonder the public is confused, especially since results reported by the media often create mixed messages. Without interpretation from an authoritative voice, confusion reigns.

Whether applying the results of the latest research as you counsel your clients or as your research team designs clinical trials, you need the ability to understand the many factors affecting nutrition science. And when talking to consumers, you must be able to provide advice based on scientific evidence even as nutrition science is evolving within an environment rife with competition for attention. Nevertheless, good scientific evidence is the foundation of good advice.

Understanding Evidence

The term *scientific evidence* is frequently used to lend validity to research results, including in the areas of food, nutrition, and dietetics. Determining the quality of evidence includes assessing multiple factors in an effort to answer the following questions:

- Were data collected ethically, safely, and in an environment that is as controlled as possible?
- Were research methods carefully and consistently applied?
- Did the research undergo a process of expert peer review?
- Was the research published in peer-reviewed journals and presented in scientific sessions?
- Who supported or funded the research?

While publication in peer-reviewed journals has been considered the gold standard for credibility of scientific information over the years, the ability to share data and papers digitally prior to review and editing—particularly in an effort to respond to emerging issues, such as the novel coronavirus pandemic—has created an opportunity for more people to analyze data sooner than the traditional process would allow. While that might lead to dissemination of unproven information, it allows for more voices to weigh in and, ultimately, may strengthen the message. As Linda Snetselaar, PhD, RDN, FAND, LD, editor-in-chief of the *Journal of the Academy of Nutrition and Dietetics,* points out in the accompanying interview, the process of reviewing papers submitted to the publication is essential to ensuring scientific rigor.

III

Linda Snetselaar, PhD, RDN, FAND, LD

Professor and Chair, Preventive Nutrition Education; Director, Nutrition Center, Department of Epidemiology, College of Public Health, University of Iowa

As editor-in-chief of the *Journal of the Academy of Nutrition and Dietetics* since 2013, Linda Snetselaar has seen the number of papers submitted for publication consideration nearly double as the influence of the journal has grown in the scientific community. "We are currently seeing more papers, including more from outside the US, that reflect new areas in the field such as metabolomics," she reports, "and we're seeing research on issues such as food insecurity in the general population as well as in relation to the COVID-19 pandemic. These submissions reflect the growing influence of our profession in scientific areas where dietitians have evidence to contribute."

The Journal of the Academy of Nutrition and Dietetics *often works with junior scientists to improve their papers, which may help them take the next step in their career.*

Snetselaar emphasizes, "We care deeply about doing all we can to help our authors succeed. Reviewers for every paper are carefully selected for their specific expertise related to the submission topic. Not only do we find reviewers who know the science, we also ask for reviews from experts who can address the clinical application of the research. The *Journal of the Academy of Nutrition and Dietetics* often works with junior scientists to improve their papers, which may help them take the next step in their career. They learn that not only is what they say valuable, but that their choice of every word also matters."

As Snetselaar notes, "Throughout the process, ensuring that each paper reflects a high degree of scientific rigor is essential."

|||

The science related to COVID-19 is a good example of the debate over science and its application. Currently, daily news briefings report "science" regarding recommended actions such as wearing masks, maintaining a social distance of at least 6 feet, and avoiding groups of more than 10 people. People asked what evidence supported these guidelines and who ensured the recommendations were credible. Communication about these recommendations was often confusing.

British journalist and businessman Matt Ridley points out in a *Wall Street Journal* article[2] that the scientific method remains the best way to determine solid evidence, despite problems such as confirmation bias, overconfidence, and political influence affecting data interpretation—not to mention all the variables involved when conducting trials.

Ridley provides a point of view that applies to our work communicating nutrition science, noting that science is better at telling us about the past and present rather than the future. For example, patients may ask about the benefit of long-term calcium on bone density. We know from past research how bone is laid down and the value of calcium in the diet early in life. Density scans can tell us the current status of our bones but not what will happen to them years or even decades into the future. Too many variables affect the outcome to be able to make definite predictions, but as we complete more research over longer time periods and learn more about individual responses to interventions, we are able to provide additional reliable counsel regarding nutrition.

Ridley also reminds us that science is a human affair. Scientists have their own views; even with solid data, they will see various theories in different ways, especially if their career has been based on these views. The only way to be sure of the reliability of a study is to examine the evidence ourselves. As food and nutrition professionals, that is our job. There are things we know (based on evidence) and things we don't know, but we need to provide counsel to the public even on topics where the science is still evolving.

Historically, experts have strived for consensus as they generated recommendations. They have come together to develop a statement reflecting their combined experiences, attitudes, and observations, but not necessarily scientific evidence. In a speech given in 2003, the late physician, writer, and producer Michael Crichton observed, "Consensus is invoked only in situations where the science is not solid enough." We need evidence, which we often don't have. Science requires only one investigator who has been able to generate genuine evidence, which means they have results that are verifiable by reference to the real world. What is relevant are reproducible results.[3] Some of the greatest scientists in history—Albert Einstein, Marie Curie, and Louis Pasteur, for example—are great precisely because they broke with traditional beliefs. We need to speak up when we find well-done studies that meet our standards and challenge the status quo while leading us to conclusions.

Gordon Guyatt, MD, distinguished professor in the Department of Clinical Epidemiology and Biostatistics at McMaster University—the birthplace of the Grading of Recommendations, Assessment, Development and Evaluation (GRADE) method for generating clinical practice guidelines—is credited with introducing the term "evidence-based medicine" in 1991 when he published an editorial in the *Annals of Internal Medicine*.[4] As cochair of the GRADE working group, Guyatt was instrumental in developing the approach that is now the standard in systematic review and development of clinical practice guidelines among more than 100 global health care organizations, including the Academy of Nutrition and Dietetics Evidence Analysis Library.

The Academy of Nutrition and Dietetics prepares members to be able to craft messages based on evidence and guides us to do so, as described in the box below.

THE ACADEMY OF NUTRITION AND DIETETICS EVIDENCE ANALYSIS LIBRARY PROVIDES RESOURCES FOR REGISTERED DIETITIAN NUTRITIONISTS

The Code of Ethics for the Nutrition and Dietetics Profession,[5] which we agree to as credentialed nutrition and dietetics practitioners, requires us to apply the best evidence from research findings to the decisions we make in our professional activities. To ensure we have access to and understanding of scientific literature in a format that can be translated into action, in 2004 the Academy of Nutrition and Dietetics established the Evidence Analysis Library (EAL). A comprehensive look at the application of evidence-based practice is provided by Raynor, Beto, and Zoellner in their article "Achieving Evidence-Based Practice in Dietetics by Using Evidence-Based Practice Guidelines" in the *Journal of the Academy of Nutrition and Dietetics*.[6] The article builds on research demonstrating the evolution of the profession's authority since the journal was launched in 1925 as the *Journal of the American Dietetic Association*.

The EAL follows now-standardized methodology used by guideline developers worldwide in all clinical practice specialties as they create systematic reviews and generate nutrition practice guidelines on a wide range of food, nutrition, and dietetics topics. Many of the Academy of Nutrition and Dietetics most requested continuing education programs offered through the Center for Lifelong Learning focus on topics related to food and nutrition research findings for which guidelines have been developed. Dietitians can refer to these guidelines as they counsel patients to develop dietary strategies during shared decision-making sessions in which they synthesize their knowledge of the research and application of the ever-evolving evidence.

In 2011, the Institute of Medicine published its *Clinical Practice Guidelines We Can Trust*, bringing more attention to the steps that lead to recommendations to ensure guidelines are reliable, useful, and actionable.[7] The rigor of clinical practice guideline development processes and proposed standards for developing trustworthy guidelines are explored relating to:

·   transparency,
·   management of conflicts of interest,
·   biases and confounders,
·   systematic reviews as related to guideline development,
·   statistical methods,
·   foundation of evidence,
·   strength of guideline recommendations,
·   articulation recommendations,
·   external reviews, and
·   updates.

In addition, "people problems" can arise. Consistency, quality control, confounding, and bias are ever-present. For example, nutrition researchers can't confirm that a study participant completes a food frequency questionnaire accurately and can't design an arm of a trial in which no one eats. While feeding studies on metabolic wards can control for these issues, that environment doesn't represent real-life conditions. This challenge is the reason many researchers believe nutrition science is one of the most complex aspects of health care.

Development of guidelines and recommendations from seemingly conflicting research can lead to controversy if evidence is not evaluated in consistent ways; however, standardization of the methodology used to review and evaluate the literature—including clear identification of the population studied, as certain groups may have been excluded from the research—informs recommendations and provides a schema for indicating how strong the evidence is. As Waleed Alhazzani, MD, MSc, associate professor in the Division of Critical Care at McMaster University and an expert in clinical practice guideline development emphatically states, "any guideline or recommendation is only as credible as its methodology." In the accompanying interviews, guidelines experts Alison Steiber, PhD, RDN, and Bram Rochwerg, MD, point out factors that practitioners should consider in applying guidelines when evidence is inconclusive.

III

Alison L. Steiber, PhD, RDN

Chief Science Officer, Academy of Nutrition and Dietetics

"Evaluating evidence is only part of the guideline development process," Alison Steiber, chief science officer at the Academy of Nutrition and Dietetics, notes as she cites many other factors that contribute to the application of nutrition guidelines. "Culture, view, perception, and access to resources are among the variables that need to be considered to yield improved outcomes when evaluating guidelines."

The majority of guidelines are not tested for their ability to be implemented, yet, in reality, barriers exist that compromise a guideline's adoptability. Applying lessons from the evolution of implementation science, dietitians have begun testing not only adoption and implementation techniques but, more importantly, considering the *effectiveness* of guidelines. Steiber asks, "Would our population be healthier if the *Dietary Guidelines for Americans* were adopted uniformly? Are they truly effective in improving the health of people who follow them?" as she considers how to measure the results of the guidelines' use.

———

"Culture, view, perception, and access to resources are among the variables that need to be considered to yield improved outcomes when evaluating guidelines."

———

"Dietitians are driving the research being done to measure the effectiveness of several of the guidelines that have been developed by the Academy of Nutrition and Dietetics Evidence Analysis Library," explains Steiber. "They've recognized the need to see if their recommendations really make a difference when put into practice. We need to know that we are providing the best care possible when we offer nutrition counseling."

I I I

Bram Rochwerg, MD, MSc, FRCPC

Juravinski Hospital ICU Site and Research Lead; Associate Professor, Department of Medicine (Division of Critical Care); Department of Health Research Methods, Evidence and Impact; GRADE Associate; GUIDE Associate; McMaster University

"It's inevitable that experts disagree," says Bram Rochwerg, an experienced methodologist who is part of McMaster University's lauded health research faculty. "Going back to the evidence base is a valuable strategy to develop consensus when writing guidelines."

When Rochwerg works with a guideline development panel trying to make a recommendation with limited evidence, he recommends contextualizing the evidence and focusing on what is agreed upon when considering the original question. Reviewing the evidence carefully and applying indirect evidence while concentrating on the most important elements of the question may yield surprising results. Voting is also a tool that can move the group toward generating a recommendation.

—

*"Going back to the evidence base
is a valuable strategy to develop
consensus when writing guidelines."*

—

As a methodologist, Rochwerg urges transparency in the guideline rationale, letting the reader know where disagreement occurred and including the dissenting opinion. Although the recommendation may be weak, it represents the best course of action given the available evidence.

I｜I

As translators of the evidence behind the dietary recommendations in the *Dietary Guidelines for Americans, 2020-2025*, we must understand the process behind the guidelines' development. For example, we know the scientific rigor reflects a strong, standardized methodology. As the current Dietary Guidelines Advisory Committee—which, as in previous editions, includes many members of the Academy of Nutrition and Dietetics—works to answer the scientific questions posed by the US Department of Agriculture and the US Department of Health and Human Services, it relies on three approaches to examine the evidence: data analysis, food pattern modeling, and systematic reviews. Each of these approaches has its own rigorous, protocol-driven methodology and plays a unique, complementary role in examining the underlying science. The type of information the advisory committee needs in order to address each scientific question determines which approach they use to review the evidence.[8]

RESEARCH UNDER SCRUTINY

Among the challenges dietitians face in translating nutrition research into the advice they provide in their daily interaction with their various publics is the fact that research, in general, faces increasing scrutiny from many fronts. While COVID-related messaging has heightened awareness of communicating evidence to the public, politics has always been a factor in presenting nutrition information. Nutrition research is, indeed, difficult to conduct because nutrition so often lacks strong, consistent evidence due to the challenges mentioned earlier. Articles and editorials about how flaws in research studies influence the interpretation of results have become more common in recent years. Controversial topics like climate change, children's vaccines, and food and nutrition are at the top of the list. Although the website reaction watch.com points out faulty design and errors in methodology and interpretation of results in published papers, even in respected journals, few people read retractions and, over time, the results stand as reported.

John Ioannidis, MD, DSc, of the Stanford Prevention Research Center and Meta-Research Innovation Center at Stanford University, is one of the most outspoken critics of scientific research. "There is increasing concern," he explains, "that most current published research findings are false. The probability that a research claim is true may depend on study power and bias, the number of other studies on the same question."[9]

Skepticism, Ioannidis explains, arises when study results cannot be reproduced due to factors such as the rush to publication, arbitrarily chosen research techniques, and the alteration of methods while a study is underway. In *The Righteous Mind*, author Jonathan Haidt, a professor at New York University, adds another dimension to irreproducibility: confirmation bias—that is, the tendency to find evidence that supports personal beliefs. It's human nature, even in science.[10] Part of our job as nutrition professionals is to identify credible and trustworthy evidence that can be used to develop guidelines and recommendations. And when we have personal views on a subject, we should make it clear that we are offering our best advice based on our own best judgment and expertise.

SORTING THE WHEAT FROM THE CHAFF

Confusion in response to health reporting has grown in tandem with the explosion of media outlets and accessibility of the information online. Results from the 2020 International Food Information Council (IFIC) Food and Health Survey indicate consumers are becoming increasingly confused about nutrition as contradictions and controversies fuel an environment of skepticism, frustration, apathy, and mistrust.[11]

Among the topics that consumers from ages 18 to 80 wanted clarified were as follows:

- Environmental sustainability: 63% of respondents say they need easier access to information about sustainability when making food choices
- Plant-based diets: half of the consumers surveyed expressed interest in a plant-based diet

- Choosing healthy foods: 23% of respondents said they actively seek out foods or follow a diet for health benefits
- Food production and food technology: 49% of respondents expressed concern about how foods are processed

As the nutrition authority, we need to be able to provide and explain the evidence to allow consumers to make healthy food choices. This includes evaluating products and recognizing healthy ingredients.

IMPROVING NUTRITION RESEARCH

Overcoming the challenges unique to nutrition research, especially consistency and confounding, presents opportunities to improve the beneficial impact of our efforts and further our authority. Our ability to use study results when developing public policy will be enhanced by ensuring study design, methodology, elimination of bias, definitions and measurements, and transparency are considered across the various research settings globally.[12] New technologies allow for improved accuracy of dietary assessments and energy intake and expenditure as well as measurement and tracking of objective biomarkers, adding to the tools available to nutrition researchers. Heightened awareness of bias in study design, recruitment, and reporting will contribute to more meaningful application of results. Integration and application of such tools and thought processes will take nutrition research to a new level.

Although people tend to react in the moment to the mixed messages generated by twists and turns around nutrition issues, most nutrition controversies have a history—deep roots that go back decades. Seemingly conflicting messages have proliferated over the years related to myriad topics including fat, caffeine, sodium, red meat, eggs, and plant-based diets. The more complex nutrition science becomes, the more complicated these issues become. And the more important nutrition becomes to the public, the more nuanced our communication strategies must become.

Writing in the journal *Advances in Nutrition Research*, Kevin Maki, PhD, president and chief science officer, Midwest Biomedical Clinical Research and Consulting, LLC, and colleagues including Penny Kris-Etherton, PhD, RDN, distinguished professor of nutrition, Penn State College of Health and Human Development, point out that although randomized control trials are the strongest study design, not all diet and health relationships can be practically or ethically evaluated that way. We are left with observational and epidemiologic studies concerning food supply and consumption and need to be clear about the scope of this research and interpret findings properly. Not all studies are longitudinal; rather, they can be snapshots of brief periods of time that may have long-term implications.[13] In the accompanying interview, Kris-Etherton considers some of the factors that contribute to success as a nutrition researcher and reflects on the research process in cardiovascular disease and the need to look forward to new evidence.

III

Penny Kris-Etherton, PhD, RDN

Penn State Clinical and Translational Science Institute (CTSI)
Evan Pugh University Professor of Nutritional Sciences
Distinguished Professor, Nutritional Sciences
Pennsylvania State University

Penny Kris-Etherton had an "aha" moment while reading about nutrition pioneer Ancel Keys' seminal research from the Seven Countries Study that showed a relationship between dietary fats and heart disease. That reaction led Kris-Etherton into a prodigious career as a research dietitian.

"Dietetics is a science-based profession," says Kris-Etherton. "We have to think like scientists and know the evidence that came before us to see where we are now and where we are going. Critical thinking and an open mind are essential as we explore what different studies and guidelines say while we work to expand the knowledge base by making new scientific discoveries. As educators, we need to teach our students to evaluate research studies carefully by reading the methods, results, and discussion sections of published scientific papers; putting these findings in context of the research evidence base being built upon; critically evaluating the differences among publications; and making the connection between food and health."

Kris-Etherton acknowledges the challenges facing researchers, such as finding funding, having a paper rejected, or, as a principal investigator, experiencing the pressure of sustaining an independent research program. This work cannot be done in isolation but benefits from interacting with colleagues in nutrition and other disciplines. "Dietitians are social people who embrace collaborations. We are known for reaching out to our colleagues to help one another." She says, "We can collaborate with people in so many different fields that span the research continuum from basic science to applied science in diverse disciplines that vary markedly."

―――

"Dietitians are social people who embrace collaborations. We are known for reaching out to our colleagues to help one another."

―――

She goes on to note, "As people who hunger for ongoing edification, we want to know the latest thinking and evidence. We explore what different organizations say, share that information with each other, and play a role in evolving new nutrition guidance. We must move forward and be committed to networking with our peers to identify collaborative opportunities, with the ultimate goal being to advance our profession."

III

Harvard TH Chan School of Public Health researchers Frank B. Hu, MD, PhD, and Walter Willett, MD, DrPH, assert that a multidisciplinary approach applied to nutritional epidemiologic studies combined with controlled feeding studies can yield robust evidence to separate myth from fact.[14] More sophisticated application of statistical analyses to increasingly large databases yields stronger evidence to inform future recommendations and policy statements.

In a viewpoint published in 2019 in the *Journal of the American Medical Association*, David S. Ludwig, MD, PhD (also of the Harvard TH Chan School of Public Health) and colleagues acknowledge the challenges inherent in nutrition research and suggest a number of steps that may improve the quality of dietary research.[15] These include:

- clarifying the minimum standards necessary for diet studies to be considered successful,
- distinguishing among study design categories and recognizing the limitations of various designs,
- acknowledging that changes or discrepancies in clinical registries of diet trials are common and may require updates to plans for data analysis,
- defining diets precisely when feasible to allow for reproducible comparisons,
- developing biomeasures of adherence,
- enhancing research infrastructure, and
- establishing best practices for communicating results.

Sifting through ever more complex and often contradictory food, health, and nutrition research to glean evidence-based, optimal, and practical applications of nutrition science requires the type of discernment dietitians are trained to deliver—the ability to continually analyze, interpret, and apply evolving research findings to create national nutrition policy while bringing sound advice to every venue where nutrition professionals work. Moving science and its application forward requires us to evaluate studies critically in the context of earlier literature. The sum of the evidence is what matters. As proponents of improved health for our clients and communities, we can look forward to obtaining more insight and greater scientific knowledge as the quality of nutrition research continues to improve.

CRAFTING AND DELIVERING MESSAGES WITH AUTHORITY

A brief look at the evolution of nutrition science shows many advances—with many more to come. Somewhere in your education you've likely been introduced to the history of nutrition. If not, be sure to check a description of Graham Lusk's classic *History of Nutrition*[16] as well as Bill Bryson's *The Body: A Guide for Occupants*.[17]

Bryson relates an interesting story about Wilbur Olin Atwater, a founder of modern food science. Following his introduction to the concept of calories while studying in Germany, Atwater devised what he called the respiratory calorimeter. In 1899, after recruiting subjects to participate in his detailed experiments, he published *The Chemical Composition of American Food Materials,* an exhaustive compilation of the caloric and nutritional values of nearly all known foods. Atwater judged the value of a food by its calorie count. Much to his surprise, he discovered that alcohol was a source of fuel. As a teetotaler and son of a clergyman, he was appalled! Nevertheless, he had to report his findings.[18]

Ultimately, most of what Atwater reported was incomplete because the role of vitamins and minerals was not yet understood, but his seminal book was a standard reference for decades. It's what we knew at the time.

In 2018, Dariush Mozaffarian, MD, DrPh, and Irwin Rosenberg, MD, of the Gerald J. and Dorothy R. Friedman School of Nutrition Science and Policy at Tufts University, and Ricardo Uauy of the London School of Hygiene and Tropical Medicine at the University of London and the Instituo de Nutricion, University of Chile, published a comprehensive article on the history of modern nutrition in the *British Medical Journal.* In this article, they presented a simplified timeline of discoveries that led to modern nutrition science, noting major themes of discovery in nutrition research since the publication of Atwater's groundbreaking work. Understanding the milestones in nutrition research and the laws of nutrition these discoveries have yielded is essential to every nutrition professional's ability to communicate the process of discovery. Themes of discovery—such as the role of vitamins in treating nutrient deficiencies, followed by the impact of single nutrients on chronic disease, followed by recognition of the significance of dietary patterns—reveal the process inherent in nutrition science.[19]

As Ken Lee, PhD, director of The Ohio State University Food Innovation Center, reminds us, science is discovery. It is never finished. We're still seeing research on vitamins and minerals that were discovered long ago, and we're still learning about interaction among nutrients, the environment, and lifestyle. Current focus on vitamin D is a prime example.

"Reporting nutrition science discoveries is a challenge because consistent evidence-based information isn't always clear," says Pamela Davis, MD, PhD, former dean, Case Western Reserve University School of Medicine. "Nutrition professionals can help reduce confusion." The growing complexity of nutrition science continues to fuel controversy and confusion among consumers and health care providers alike. Escalating health care costs as well as advances in medical science and technology compel us to look at new models for prevention and treatment. Meanwhile, public health leaders, advocates for food access, environmentalists, food technologists, economists, and agriculture experts all warn us that climate change, population growth, and shifting demographics are threatening the world's food supply, thus undermining the nutrition and health of future generations. Responding intelligently to these challenges requires research and an understanding of how to interpret findings. It requires each of us to be that communicator and authority who conveys understanding of the evidence and offers the best advice we know at the time. In the accompanying interview, Mary Lee Chin, MS, RDN, an early Academy of Nutrition and Dietetics spokesperson, offers insight from her career addressing controversial issues as a nutrition communicator unafraid to stand up for the best science.

I|I

Mary Lee Chin, MS, RDN

Nutrition Edge Communications

"Being part of the Academy of Nutrition and Dietetics spokesperson program was crucial to my career," states 2020 Lenna

Frances Cooper Memorial Lecturer award-winner Mary Lee Chin, MS, RDN. She adds, "I have always had a love of communication science and, as a dietitian, I have the opportunity to use those skills to help educate the public in so many different areas. As an Academy of Nutrition and Dietetics spokesperson, I had a chance to expand beyond clinical settings to many other audiences."

———

"In a time of nutrition misinformation among the public, learning how people make decisions, really listening to their beliefs, and being responsive while remaining open and engaged allows you to find common ground so your messages are trusted and accepted."

———

Examples Chin cites include crafting messages on topics as varied as public health, the food supply chain, industry, environmental science, waste management, and research. "In a time of nutrition misinformation among the public, learning how people make decisions, really listening to their beliefs, and being responsive while remaining open and engaged allows you to find common ground so your messages are trusted and accepted," says Chin.

Recalling her experiences in clinical settings, Chin points out that dietitians operate as part of a team. From collaborating with physicians, nurse educators, psychologists, and social workers to determine how to help a rebellious teenager manage their diabetes, to engaging with community leaders, food producers, schools, and churches to ensure communities have access to nutritious food, dietitians need to demonstrate cultural literacy to ensure their messages will be considered relevant and trustworthy. "We need to be informed, aware, and engaged in society as a whole to reach our audience, wherever they are," Chin advises.

⁂

You probably are well aware of the controversial topics in nutrition these days; clients, patients, friends, and family often ask about the latest research on popular diets or food recommendations they see posted on social media. We hate not being able to answer questions posed to us. In fact, we know how to evaluate these studies to determine their credibility. But in addition to knowing the science, we need the communication skills to ensure our messages are understood and applied by our audience.

The Alan Alda Center for Communicating Science teaches students—including scientists and health professionals—how to communicate complex topics in clear, vivid, and engaging ways. A statement from the Center (sponsored by renowned actor and lifetime science buff Alan Alda) explains that effective communication happens when we listen and connect. It happens when we use empathy. Communication is headed for success when we pay more attention to what the other person is understanding rather than focusing solely on what we want to say.[20] The Center's approach to communication has always impressed me, and I think it is relevant to us as we design our own communications philosophy. First and foremost, we should strive to listen and connect.

Building on that foundation, Barbara Mayfield, MS, RDN, of Nutrition Communicator, LLC, and editor of *Communicating Nutrition: The Authoritative Guide*, offers five tips for communicating science[21]:

1. Understand the nature of research.
2. Interpret research accurately.
3. Create context.
4. Beware of bias.
5. Communicate findings clearly.

One of the simplest yet most effective communications models comes from the late Bernadine Healy, MD, the first female head of the National Institutes of Health and chief architect of the Women's Health Initiative. A brilliant communicator, Healy served as dean of the College of Public Health at The Ohio State University, director of the Red Cross, and a health editor and a columnist for *US News & World Report,* and she was a respected commentator in news media.

Healy's three-part model became a mantra for many communicators, whether they were giving a talk to business colleagues or a presentation to dietitians. When communicating information, especially when that information is controversial, tell your audience:

- Here is what we know.
- Here is what we don't know.
- Based on that knowledge (and Healy's own well-recognized authority), here is what to do.

In addition, thought leaders—defined by Keith Carlson as "keenly intelligent, forward-thinking individuals who see the realities of the current state of affairs in their area of influence and strive to foment change [and] visualize, create or inspire new solutions"—serve as role models and inspiration as we demonstrate authority in our daily professional lives.[22] Thought leaders are acutely aware of the way the wind is blowing and able to predict what will arrive on the next zephyr. Whether their leadership is self proclaimed or identified by colleagues, thought leaders are the people who inspire us to step up to exert our authority and influence to effect change.

In *The Workshop and the World: What Ten Thinkers Can Teach Us About Science and Authority*, philosopher and science historian Robert Crease reminds us that scientific authority has been embodied in thought leaders since people such as Francis Bacon, Galileo Galilei, and Descartes first described scientific authority as an addition to spiritual and secular authority in the fifteenth century.[23]

Given the nature of nutrition research and the public's hunger for data, the demand for credible interpretation of nutrition science will continue to grow. We have the skills needed to evaluate the veracity of research and to judge which findings to include in our messages to various audiences. As individuals and as a profession, we need to be certain our credibility and basis in science are not compromised as we work to meet the demands of the global public. Things we can do to demonstrate our authority include reading carefully, understanding research methods, drawing on colleagues' areas of expertise, and providing advice on what we can do as evidence evolves.

REFERENCES

1. Krauthammer C. Opinion: The myth of "settled science." The Washington Post website; February 20, 2014. Accessed October 21, 2021. www.washingtonpost .com/opinions/charles-krauthammer-the-myth-of-settled-science/2014/02/20 /c1f8d994-9a75-11e3-b931-0204122c514b_story.html

2. Ridley M. What the pandemic has taught us about science. The Wall Street Journal website; October 10, 2020. Accessed October 21, 2021. www.wsj.com /articles/what-the-pandemic-has-taught-us-about-science-11602255638

3. Crichton M. Aliens cause global warming. Michelin Lecture presented at CalTech Institute of Technology. January 17, 2003. Accessed October 21, 2021. https://stephenschneider.stanford.edu/Publications/PDF_Papers /Crichton2003.pdf

4. Guyatt GH. Evidence-based medicine. ACP J Club. 1991;114(suppl 2):A-16.

5. Academy of Nutrition and Dietetics, Commission on Dietetic Registration. Code of Ethics for the Nutrition and Dietetics Profession. June 1, 2018. Accessed October 21, 2021. www.eatrightpro.org/-/media/eatrightpro-files /career/code-of-ethics/coeforthenutritionanddieteticsprofession.pdf

6. Raynor HA, Beto JA, Zoellner J. Achieving evidence-based practice in dietetics by using evidence-based practice guidelines. J Acad Nutr Diet. 2020 May;120(5):751-756. doi:10.1016/j.jand.2019.10.011

7. Institute of Medicine. Clinical Practice Guidelines We Can Trust. National Academies Press; 2011.

8. Dietary Guidelines Advisory Committee. Scientific Report of the 2020 Dietary Guidelines Advisory Committee: Advisory Report to the Secretary of Agriculture and the Secretary of Health and Human Services. US Department of Agriculture, Agricultural Research Service, Washington, DC; 2020. Accessed October 21, 2021. www.dietaryguidelines.gov/2020-advisory-committee-report

9. Ioannidis JPA. Why most published research findings are false. PLoS Med. 2005;2(8):e124. doi:10.1371/journal.pmed.0020124

10. Haidt J. The Righteous Mind: Why Good People are Divided by Politics and Religion. Pantheon Books; 2012

11. 2020 Food & Health Survey. International Food Information Council; June 9, 2020. Accessed October 21, 2021. https://ific.org/wp-content/uploads/2021 /02/2020-IFIC-Annual-Report.pdf

12. Gardner, CD, Crimarco A, Landry MJ, Fielding-Singh P. Nutrition study design issues—important issues for interpretation. *Am J Health Promotion.* 2020;34:951-954. doi:10.1177/0890117120960580d

13. Maki KC, Slavin JL, Rains TM, Kris-Etherton PM. Limitations of observational evidence: implications for evidence-based dietary recommendations. *Advances in Nutrition.* 2014;5:7-15. doi:10.3945/an.113.004929

14. Hu FB, Willett WC. Current and future landscape of nutritional epidemiologic research. *JAMA.* 2018;320:2073-2074.

15. Ludwig DS, Ebbeling CB, Heymsfield SB: Improving the quality of dietary research. *JAMA.* 2019. doi:10.1001/jama.2019.11169

16. Striker C. Graham Lusk and his contributions to the science of nutrition. *Diabetes.* 1953 May-Jun;2(3):242-3. doi:10.2337/diab.2.3.242

17. Bryson B. *The Body: A Guide for Occupants.* Doubleday; 2019.

18. Atwater WO, Bryant AP. *The Chemical Composition of American Food Materials.* US Government Printing Office; 1899.

19. Mozaffarian D, Rosenberg I, Uauy R. History of modern nutrition science—implications for current research, dietary guidelines, and food policy. *BMJ.* 2018;361:K239.

20. Science Counts, Alan Alda Center for Communicating Science. Assessing scientists' willingness to engage in science communication. Accessed October 30, 2021. https://sciencecounts.org/wp-content/uploads/2019/06/Assessing -Scientist-Willingness-to-Engage-in-Science-Communication.pdf

21. Mayfield B, ed. *Communicating Nutrition: The Authoritative Guide.* Academy of Nutrition and Dietetics; 2020.

22. Carlson K. Healthcare thought leaders: who they are, and why we need them. *Multibriefs: Exclusive website.* March 5, 2020. Accessed October 21, 2021. https://exclusive.multibriefs.com/content/healthcare-thought-leaders-who-they -are-and-why-we-need-them/healthcare-administration

23. Crease RP. *The Workshop and the World: What Ten Thinkers Can Teach Us About Science and Authority.* W.W. Norton and Company; 2019.

SECTION THREE

New Frontiers: Applying Research to Achieve Our Vision

———————————————

Delving into the future is a formidable task. Many opportunities are evolving in various areas for registered dietitian nutritionists (RDNs) to achieve success in new roles, but no clear steps or checklists exist to show the way. Regardless of your area of practice, meeting the future depends on a deep understanding of the profession and a plan to find the gaps where RDNs can add value and offer solutions to a problem.

Communicating with up-and-coming RDNs who have already distinguished themselves in the profession has reinforced my belief that opportunities are vast for our profession. Luis Gonzalez, MS, RDN, an account coordinator at Eat Well Global and leader of the Academy of Nutrition and Dietetics member interest group Latinos and Hispanics in Dietetics and

Nutrition (LAHIDAN) states that "RDNs are capable and qualified to work in just about any arena where food is present." As an RDN in communications, Gonzalez sees roles for more RDNs, especially underrepresented RDNs, working in-house with brands as well as in agencies to ensure food work is managed by professionals with a background in food and nutrition. Gonzalez emphasizes that dietitians need to be in front of the public more frequently, particularly via major media organizations such as CNN and *The New York Times.*

In fact, it was seeing Carolyn O'Neil, MS, RDN, on CNN's new segment On the Menu that influenced Marie Allsopp, DrPH, RD, LD, CHES, clinical assistant professor, Department of Nutrition Science at Purdue University and first Academy of Nutrition and Dietetics Foundation Diversity and Inclusion Fellow to see a future for herself in the profession of dietetics. As she earned multiple academic degrees and gained clinical insight, Allsopp was and still is a leader in local and Academy of Nutrition and Dietetics-wide organizations. She sees opportunities for RDNs to embrace our multicultural and multilingual society and, as a result of the pandemic, increase our remote work in wellness and weight control. Allsopp also believes increasing our profession's presence in media and social media—perhaps in partnership with government agencies, such as the FDA and USDA, and restaurants and supermarkets that use the services of corporate dietitians—would reinforce the profession's authority. As an Academy of Nutrition and Dietetics Foundation Fellow, Allsopp is working to identify and overcome barriers that students of diverse cultures and backgrounds face in pursuing a career in nutrition and dietetics, and she is leading the Academy of Nutrition and Dietetics Foundation program to support students and practitioners in overcoming obstacles in recruitment, education, and advancement.

The attitudes toward the profession and the thought rising leaders have given to strengths and weaknesses of our profession can only strengthen the dietitians' influence on public health and challenges related to food and nutrition in our society. Regardless of your career path, there is a great need for qualified professionals working on the prevention and treatment of chronic disease. The Centers for Medicaid and Medicare Services (CMS) provides a list of 21 of the most common chronic diseases; many of these are affected by diet and nutrition and, therefore, point to a strong, ongoing demand for dietitians.[1] In fact, almost all chronic diseases speak to a relationship between nutrition and health. This is likely to increase as the US population ages and adopts an increasingly sedentary lifestyle.

The National Health Council estimates approximately 133 million people—representing 40% of the population—are affected by at least one chronic disease, and that number is on the rise.[2] And the Centers for Disease Control and Prevention (CDC) estimates that six of 10 Americans suffer from a chronic disease, while four of those six people have two or more of these conditions.[3] Diabetes is the fastest growing chronic disease, with more than 100 million adults with diabetes in the United States.[3] The top three chronic diseases in the United States—heart disease, cancer, and diabetes—all require our professional expertise. According to the CDC, these three diseases are also the leading drivers of the nation's $3.8 trillion annual health care costs.[3]

Opportunities abound for us to apply our knowledge and skills to improve the health of society. That is our mission as a profession, and it is reflected in our work to help feed Americans and help people facing food insecurity. Feeding America data illuminate the scope of the problem and the number of people in need of dietetic and nutrition services.[4] For example, more than 42 million people may experience food insecurity, including 13 million children; 35 million people in the United States experienced hunger in 2019, and that number only increased during the COVID-19 pandemic. Many households that experience food insecurity do not qualify for federal nutrition programs. While many innovative programs are underway, these facts demonstrate that we have multiple opportunities to demonstrate our creativity and dedication to helping people improve their health and wellbeing. We need to explore how to help and position our profession in diverse settings where our knowledge, authority, and expertise contribute to a healthier world.

When the Academy of Nutrition and Dietetics began planning its centennial anniversary, leaders recognized that the time was ideal to reexamine their current plan and take bold steps to look at the future and bring focus to the Academy of Nutrition and Dietetics Second Century priorities. They convened a Nutrition Impact Summit that included relevant experts from diverse fields around the world as well as past, present, and future leaders from all segments of the Academy of Nutrition and Dietetics. The attendees explored innovative solutions to today's unique public health challenges and identified opportunities for partners to collaborate and stimulate improvements in national and global health through food and nutrition.[5] Although designed to guide the Academy of Nutrition and Dietetics into the future, the Academy of Nutrition and Dietetics Second Century vision applies to individual RDNs and should be considered and adopted to help identify new ventures and provide a platform for action.

The Nutrition Impact Summit helped create a new vision and mission for the Academy of Nutrition and Dietetics that reflect the profession's global presence. These statements act as guidelines as we chart our future in the profession and strengthen our commitment to world health.

Vision: A world where all people thrive through the transformative power of food and nutrition

Mission: Accelerate improvements in global health and well-being through food and nutrition

I decided to look at two paths that should be important to all RDNs, regardless of where they work: the food system and information technology. Casting a wide net around the food system and information technology captures opportunities for all RDNs. Research is focused on the personal approach to health care, and government and health care practitioners are recognizing advances that can be made there. First, let's take a closer look into the food system, which is an area of interest for many professional groups.

THE FOOD SYSTEM

Working within the food supply chain (agriculture practices, food processing, packaging, distribution, and retail) requires us to understand the pertinent issues that enhance our authority. Clients and consumers are going to demand more of us as they seek information about the food system—for example, where and how food is grown, processed, and distributed. Regardless of whether we provide traditional services or focus on emerging approaches, exploring opportunities within the food system is essential.

For example, Andie Lee Gonzalez, PhD, MPH, RDN, LD, FAND is on the front lines in retail markets along the border between Texas and Mexico. She provides insight to what it takes to be in retail and what knowledge is required.

⏐⏐⏐

Andie Lee Gonzalez, PhD, MPH, RDN, LD, FAND

Abbott, Pediatric Medical Science Liaison; formerly H-E-B Grocery Company

"The sky's the limit!" exclaims Andie Gonzalez, who served as 2021–2022 chair of the Academy of Nutrition and Dietetics Latinos and Hispanics in Dietetics and Nutrition Member Interest Group. "There's lots of opportunity in non-traditional roles for dietitians, but you have to be open to the possibilities, connect with other people, step up, and take the risk. You never know who's watching."

Gonzalez heard of a job opening for a dietitian in Texas, her home state, at the H-E-B grocery chain. After a thorough long-distance interview, Gonzalez traveled from Michigan, where she had attended Michigan State University, to H-E-B headquarters in San Antonio for a final in-person interview. "I literally drove up in my U-Haul," she remembers. "I got the job and worked for the company for 7 years."

―――――

"There's lots of opportunity in non-traditional roles for dietitians, but you have to be open to the possibilities, connect with other people, step up, and take the risk."

―――――

Gonzalez began as an in-store dietitian. After about 4 years on the job, she transitioned into sales and marketing related to H-E-B's health and wellness efforts, where she creates relationships with key stakeholders, such as wellness programs and doctors' offices, to promote H-E-B's nutrition services.

Gonzalez says measuring the impact of your services is a challenge when working as an RDN in retail. "For a program to survive," she says, "it must show a return on investment, whether it be hard (money) or soft (reputation, loyalty, trust, etc). That's why a business education is so important for nutrition professionals in any setting."

Of all her accomplishments, Gonzalez is most proud of her nutrition services work in the Rio Grande Valley, in places like her hometown, Palmview. "Ninety percent of the people who live in Texas border towns are Hispanic or Hispanic-American. It's a unique culture," she says. In 2021, Gonzalez began work as a pediatric medical science liaison for Abbott where she continues her nutrition journey and strives to push the needle forward.

As the United Nations High Level Panel of Experts (HLPE) on Food Security and Nutrition explains, "food systems gather all the elements and activities that relate to the production, processing, distribution, preparation, and consumption of food, and the output of these activities including socioeconomic, sociocultural, nutrition and health, and environmental outcomes" (see Figure 1).[6]

Food systems are not linear; rather, they are a series of complex feedback loops. No one food system is "best," nor can one model address all needs and all circumstances. While varying in complexity, every food system comprises subsystems. Eileen Kennedy, PhD, RDN, a member of the HLPE, often speaks to the panel about the value of nutrition professionals in the multilayered food system, offering a comprehensive way to consider where we are and where we're going. The HLPE breaks the food system into four components—food supply chains, food environments, individual factors, and consumer behavior—all of which interact to influence diet, nutrition, and health outcomes.[6]

Making our mark in the food system requires us to grasp the whole picture, understand the complex issues that face the entire system, and provide knowledgeable advice and services relevant to solving problems and making recommendations. That is what it takes to be an authority, and this is where opportunities arise.

So where do we start to carve out our role? Reports from government bodies around the world provide some guidance. For example, the United Nations Sustainable Development Goals (SDGs) (see Figure 2) commit UN members to "end hunger, achieve food security and improved nutrition, and promote sustainable agriculture." They provide a powerful framework to guide decisions on policies and budgets by governments, the private sector, and civil society.[7]

Sustainability is a word seen frequently in government reports and academic writing. The word has multiple definitions; this one, from the University of California Los Angeles, is most useful in our context[8]:

The integration of environmental health, social equity and economic vitality in order to create thriving, healthy, diverse and resilient communities for this generation and generations to come. The practice of sustainability recognizes how these issues are interconnected and requires a systems approach and an acknowledgment of complexity. Sustainable practices support ecological, human, and economic health and vitality. Sustainability presumes that resources are finite and should be used conservatively and wisely with a view to long-term priorities and consequences of the ways in which resources are used.

Sustainability issues speak to RDNs. Marie Spiker, PhD, RDN, was an Academy of Nutrition and Dietetics Foundation Fellow who focused on agriculture issues for the profession. These issues, especially sustainability, are central in the RDN's scope of responsibility.

Figure 1 Conceptual framework of food systems for diets and nutrition

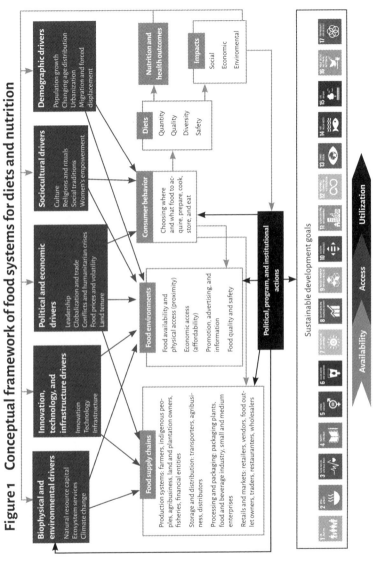

Source: HLPE. 2017. *Nutrition and Food Systems: A Report by the High Level Panel of Experts on Food Security and Nutrition.* www.fao.org/3/i7846e/i7846e.pdf. Reproduced with permission.

Figure 2   Sustainable development goals

   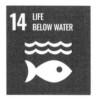

Source: HLPE. 2017. *Nutrition and Food Systems: A Report by the High Level Panel of Experts on Food Security and Nutrition.* www.fao.org/3/i7846e/i7846e.pdf. Reproduced with permission.

III

Marie Spiker, PhD, MSPH, RDN

Assistant Professor, Nutritional Sciences Program; Core Faculty, Food Systems, Nutrition, and Health; University of Washington's School of Public Health

Marie Spiker is an assistant professor in the University of Washington School of Public Health. As an Academy of Nutrition and Dietetics Foundation Fellow (2018–2020), she led the Academy of Nutrition and Dietetics strategic initiatives to empower nutrition and dietetics professionals to be leaders in sustainable, resilient, and healthy food and water systems.

———

"In other words, the food system is about much more than food. It's a microcosm of the world."

———

"Not long ago," Spiker observes, "the food system was a behind-the-scenes concept. Now, however, it's become a critical model for understanding the complex and synergistic way food moves from farm to production to distribution to the kitchen table. In other words, the food system is about much more than food. It's a microcosm of the world."

Spiker reports that University of Washington students from various disciplines including policy, engineering, technology, forestry, and urban design are attracted to studying the food system. There's enough interest, in fact, that the university has established an undergraduate major in food systems, nutrition, and health.

Some dietitians may not fully grasp how the food system affects their work. "A better perspective might be how their work affects the food system," Spiker notes, adding that all food and nutrition professionals should have a certain level of awareness about the food system because nutrition is involved in every component. "But nutrition is only one piece of the puzzle," Spiker explains. "To fully participate in the whole system, we must learn about the other stakeholders and their goals."

Spiker notes that despite so much diversity in their professional roles today, dietitians "are on the same page" and share a common thread—their role in the food system.

III

Food safety and the prevention of food waste are two issues squarely in the RDN's wheelhouse. To see the food system as an integrated whole, however, we need to see the relationships among all its parts. Spiker reminds us that issues around food fall into our area of expertise and are our responsibility. Being an authority requires us to participate in a manner that shows we grasp the complexity of the system.

Timing is everything when it comes to making an impact. You may recall the United Nations (UN) announced a major focus on nutrition—another key global initiative. The UN Decade of Action on Nutrition (2016–2025) emphasizes the importance of joint efforts among UN agencies, academia, civil society, and the private sector. Sustainable food systems for healthful diets is one of the plan's pillars.[9] This is a global call for our engagement. We need to understand the landscape in order to offer effective ways to improve the nutritional health of all people. But where do we stand with the UN? What steps are most urgent and critical? Where and how can RDNs engage? Opportunities to demonstrate our value exist, but where do we start? Winona Bynum, RDN, PMP, and communications specialist David Mitchell offer some advice on how to engage at the local level in support the UN Decade of Action on Nutrition.

I | I

Winona Bynum, RDN, PMP

Executive Director, Detroit Food Policy Council

How did a software project manager working for Hewlett Packard (HP) supporting General Motors (GM) become a registered dietitian and executive director of the Detroit Food Policy Council? "I had an 'aha!' moment," says Winona Bynum. "My diet was not very good, and I wasn't feeling that great. My manager at HP suggested I look at my diet." As Bynum changed how she ate, she started to feel better. "I learned that people don't know the power of food—how it works and the science behind it," she explains. Thus began her second career.

―――

"I learned that people don't know the power of food—how it works and the science behind it."

―――

In 2010, Bynum enrolled in the dietetics program at Wayne State University, graduated in 2012, and took her credentialing exam in 2013. After doing community organizing for the Fair Food Network, Bynum went on to manage youth and nutrition programs for Gleaners Community Food Bank of Southeastern Michigan. She studied public health at Emory University. In 2015, she joined the Detroit Food Policy Council (DFPC) as its executive director.

The DFPC is an education, advocacy, and policy organization that is one of the more than 300 food policy councils connected through the Johns Hopkins Center for a Livable Future. Unlike most food councils, which come out of government, the DFPC is the result of grassroots community action. It is a free-standing, 23-member, nonprofit advisory board that includes representatives from various sectors of the food system, at-large representatives, a youth representative, and government representatives from the mayor's office, city council, and health department. "Board members work together to try to better understand the needs of each sector with the aim of creating a sustainable and equitable food system that serves everyone in the community," Bynum notes. "What's good for one group isn't necessarily good for all."

Bynum, the 2021–2022 chair of the Academy of Nutrition and Dietetics National Organization of Blacks in Dietetics and Nutrition (NOBIDAN), says that her experience in business has been very helpful to her as the DFPC's executive director. That, plus the fact that she is perhaps the only US dietitian in such a position, makes Bynum a pioneer and a model of what can be done at the intersection of public health and food systems. When students reach out to her, Bynum encourages them to use their knowledge to elevate the profession and educate others on the power of food.

I‖I

David Mitchell

Founder and President, Patients For Affordable Drugs

As a communications specialist with more than 30 years' experience managing a cause-oriented public policy firm in Washington, DC, David Mitchell has successfully led campaigns that have reduced teen smoking, increased use of seatbelts, fought drunk driving, and improved child health and safety. In his retirement, he is now serving as founder and president of the advocacy group Patients For Affordable Drugs.

———

Mitchell emphasized that establishing a professional curriculum that is responsive to cultural factors and focuses on the complete food cycle—from what food is planted to what is available in various locations around the globe—is crucial to creating a healthy public.

———

When asked about opportunities for dietitians to shape health for the future, Mitchell firmly recommends marshaling the enthusiasm and expertise demonstrated by members on the front lines to work for education and policy changes where health outcomes can be measured. Mitchell emphasized that establishing a professional curriculum that is responsive to cultural factors and focuses on the complete food cycle—from what food is planted to what is available in various locations around the globe—is crucial to creating a healthy public. Dietitians can provide their knowledge and authority along all parts of the arc of that process.

"Find the dietitian who is ahead of the curve, who can connect where something is happening to make it bigger," advises Mitchell. "Advocate for education and policy through the strength of the Academy of Nutrition and Dietetics as an organizational driving force. This also provides an opportunity for younger people to come in at the local level and make a name for themselves as they champion their vision for improvement."

III

The Academy of Nutrition and Dietetics Foundation has developed a framework for action that identifies five entry points related to sustainable food and water systems:

1. Shape and deliver dietary guidance.
2. Improve security of food, nutrition, and water.
3. Align food production and nutrition.
4. Optimize supply chains and food environments.
5. Reduce waste.

These points must be developed and used to leverage the strength within individual practice settings and as part of multi-sectored collaborations. This work requires coordination between the areas of education and training, research, practice, and policy.[10]

In their *Journal of the Academy of Nutrition and Dietetics* article, "Food System Sustainability: An Academy of Nutrition and

Dietetics Advocacy Priority," Jeanne Blankenship, MS, RDN, and Robyn Smith Brown, MBA, RD, LDN, remind us that "legislative and regulatory initiatives are a key factor in aligning sustainability across multiple sectors and generating buy-in from environmental, government, health, and nutrition stakeholders. The [Academy of Nutrition and Dietetics Foundation] framework for action has set the stage for future policy considerations and reaffirmed the Academy of Nutrition and Dietetics current initiatives."[11] Partnerships are created through these collaborations and open doors to dialogue and solutions to improve nutritional health.

As Francesco Branca, director of the World Health Organization Department of Nutrition for Health and Development, stated regarding a report on malnutrition published in *The Lancet*[12,13]:

We are facing a new nutrition reality. We can no longer characterize countries as low-income and undernourished or high-income and only concerned with obesity. All forms of malnutrition have a common denominator—food systems that fail to provide all people with healthy, safe, affordable, and sustainable diets. Changing this will require action across food systems, from production and processing, through trade and distribution, pricing, marketing, and labeling, to consumption and waste.

Branca refers to a set of double-duty actions that simultaneously prevents or reduces the risk of nutritional deficiencies leading to underweight, wasting, and stunting; micronutrient deficiencies; and obesity or noncommunicable diseases with the same intervention, including new agricultural and food system policies with healthy diets as their primary goal. These recommendations are a call for us to understand and act as the voice of authority.

At a 2014 consensus conference organized as part of the Academy of Nutrition and Dietetics international strategic plan, Academy of Nutrition and Dietetics leaders took a hard look at the intersection of agriculture and health to identify areas where food and nutrition professionals can make a difference in the food system.[14] The steps identified included:

- promoting agricultural innovation and sustainable farming techniques;
- advocating for safe, nutritious, and efficient food processing, packaging, storage, and transportation;
- collaborating with retailers to increase access to nutrient-dense foods and encourage healthy options;
- using evidence-based nutrition information to teach consumers healthy eating behaviors;
- serving as nutritional liaisons between policy makers, science, and the public on legislation such as the Farm Bill and the Child Nutrition and WIC Reauthorization Act;
- using evidence-based clinical and community nutrition knowledge; and
- promoting or engaging in strategies for energy and water conservation and waste minimization.

These are suggested areas that require study and engagement to realize opportunities. Who better than food and nutrition professionals to develop training and standards of practice to promote food and nutrition security worldwide?

Regardless of our level of engagement in food-system issues, we all need to help consumers understand what is known and what is not known, based on science. The AgriNutrition Edge Report, a blog by Marianne Smith Edge, MS, RDN, LD, FAND, delivers sound knowledge and communicates messages that can be helpful in practice.

I‖I

Marianne Smith Edge, MS, RDN, LD, FAND

Founder and Principal, The AgriNutrition Edge

As a sixth-generation farm owner, Marianne Smith Edge didn't need to look far to see the connection between what is in the fields and what is on consumers' plates. With lessons from her youth on a dairy farm added to her education in the science of nutrition and dietetics, Smith Edge has built a strong brand by applying her critical thinking and nutrition knowledge in various positions—such as a consultant dietitian in health care facilities, as senior vice president at the International Food Information Council, and as president of the Academy of Nutrition and Dietetics. As consumer and professional interest in sustainability and food systems has grown, Smith Edge has recognized that taking her experience back to her roots was the logical next step in her career.

Messages on her popular blog clearly demonstrate Smith Edge's ability to communicate clear, science-based messages on controversial topics. "I can speak about agriculture with a nutrition focus," she explains. "By combining my experience in food, nutrition, agriculture, and consumer behavior, I can work with groups who want to provide safe, accessible food that meets nutritional needs in various settings. As dietitians, we can work in areas, such as food technology, sustainability, food insecurity, and food waste. By applying the same critical thinking skills and evidence-based science to food systems as [we do] to clinical dietetics, we can be a key player in this space."

―――

"We have the science background to provide insights into all aspects of the system to enhance food, agriculture, and consumer experiences."

―――

Smith Edge believes that because food and nutrition professionals recognize the complexity and intricacies of food systems globally, they can clarify concepts around local sourcing, agriculture production, and plant-based eating. "We have the science background to provide insights into all aspects of the system to enhance food, agriculture, and consumer experiences," Smith Edge notes.

I ‖ I

The food system can be a healthy, equitable engine for local economic growth. A strong area for market expansion for food and nutrition professionals, the food system provides a foundation for thinking differently about our contributions to health, sustainability, and food justice and forces us to see how its various aspects influence what we say and do. Achieving success requires partnerships and engaging with other professional groups. Building collaborations is essential to improving the health of the world.

INFORMATION TECHNOLOGY

Like food systems, information technology (IT) is critical and will remain so in the future. Information technology affords new opportunities for nutrition and dietetics professionals and influences how we practice and how we position ourselves as nutrition authorities.

In 2020, nearly one in five Americans was using a mobile health monitoring device or app related to diet and food consumption, exercise and physical activity, or overall health. Nearly all of these users reported feeling more aware of their health status, and two-thirds said the device or app has led them to make healthy changes in their life.[15] This is just the beginning. Thanks to electronic health records, telehealth, big-data analytics, and artificial intelligence, consumers have more control over key aspects of their health, and medical professionals (including food and nutrition professionals) have more discrete information available to care for individual patients and provide consumer advice.

Google is a major force in the technology space. Chavanne Hanson, MPH, RDN, a Google employee, describes the fast pace of the company and the many dimensions of the technology fields in which food and nutrition professionals can find opportunities and create value.

I|I

Chavanne Hanson, MPH, RDN

Food Choice Architect and Nutrition Manager, Global Food Team, Google

In describing her career path, Chavanne Hanson of Google's Global Food Team says, "It's all about people. Chance meetings can turn into solid relationships that open doors in unexpected places. Push yourself to connect with others and spend time getting to know people. Those 'soft skills' are often vital."

———

"It's all about people. Chance meetings can turn into solid relationships that open doors in unexpected places."

———

Having transitioned from working as a research dietitian in public health, to clinical dietetics, then to the culinary world (where she worked for Chef Graham Kerr), and then to global public affairs at Nestlé, Hanson recalls every experience as a stepping-stone toward her current position at Google, where she is engaged with teams that provide healthy meals to Google employees across the world. Increasingly, colleagues call upon Hanson to share her perspective on issues all dietitians are concerned about, such as sustainability and food waste.

Being open to new ideas and opportunities enabled Hanson to apply the wide range of knowledge that she acquired in her RDN education. "I'm a connector," she explains. "Being able to put the right people together is essential. Looking at supply-chain architecture through the lens of a dietitian emphasizes the wide range of professional opportunities that are evolving in our profession. No one can know everything, so being able to bring in experts via connections made through the Academy of Nutrition and Dietetics, its Dietetic Practice Groups, and culinary and agriculture organizations is so valuable."

Hanson emphasizes that challenges abound, due to how much dietitians need to know in many areas. "You can never do too much background reading," she advises. "Be well read, be prepared, and listen. Knowing what questions to ask is the mark of a well-curated professional."

III

Advances in information technology happen quickly, which can make it hard to keep up and even harder to foresee future developments, tools, and applications unimaginable today. But we know the future will provide us with more innovative ways to use information technology to strengthen our role as providers of food, nutrition, and dietetics services. For now, let's consider some things we are already doing, starting with telehealth, and also look at the importance of big data, artificial intelligence, and how these innovations affect personal or precision nutrition.

Telehealth

Telehealth and *telemedicine* are terms used interchangeably to describe the provision of health care services and information via telecommunication technology.[16] While its value and visibility have been heightened by the COVID-19 pandemic, telehealth had already been identified as an important, cost-effective, and convenient tool for dietitians to use in delivering reliable nutrition information, education, counseling, and monitoring in ways that expand the reach of the profession. As Medicare, insurers, regulators, and other stakeholders have recognized the medium's ability to provide increased health care delivery via an internet connection, opportunities have increased for dietitians to offer their services and be reimbursed using this expanding delivery mechanism.

The Academy of Nutrition and Dietetics has recognized the potential of telehealth in our practice for many years and includes resources on the Academy of Nutrition and Dietetics website. In 2020, the Academy of Nutrition and Dietetics convened a Telehealth Task Force to develop a formal policy stance to increase access to medical nutrition therapy and foster the visibility of members who provide telehealth services. In April 2021, the Academy of Nutrition and Dietetics board adopted a five-part stance on telehealth policy that addresses such issues as licensure, funding, access, equity, and research.[17]

While outcomes data on the effectiveness of telehealth have yet to be measured, early studies on patient experiences (to assess patient satisfaction during virtual visits) indicate virtual visits are comparable to in-person visits and support the value and acceptance of such visits.[18] Assessments of technology and patient-clinician engagement as well as comparison to in-person visit outcomes are research opportunities for dietitians to generate valuable information on expansion of this care-delivery method.

What Makes Data "Big"?

All technological advances are dependent on the quality and quantity of data. Data can come from many sources, including wearable technologies, such as pedometers and heart-rate monitors; Wifi-connected appliances; smartphones and cameras; social media platforms; computer gaming; sensors in the home and environment around us; tracked online purchasing; retail loyalty programs; credit and debit cards; browsing histories; insurance companies' records; medical records (within HIPAA regulations); industrial and agricultural technologies (eg, chemical and livestock monitoring)—and the list goes on.

Generally recognized components of Big Data include:

- **Volume:** The amount of data collected, stored, and curated.
- **Velocity:** The speed with which data are collected. In agriculture and nutrition, Big Data offer an opportunity for near-real-time analyses and decisions made based on weather patterns, nutritional status, and agricultural production.

- **Variety:** The type of data collected. The more variety within a data set, the more robust and potentially meaningful the data become for a specific application, such as agriculture and nutrition.
- **Veracity:** The reliability of the data source. Good decisions require good data.
- **Value:** The insights that are generated must be based on accurate data and lead to measurable improvements.[19]

Big Data help researchers develop evidence and developers create useful software applications. Subsequently, information entered in applications adds data to the pool. As censoring technology and the number of smartphones increase, so do the data these tools generate. Joyce Gilbert, PhD, RDN, analyzes Big Data to grow the Association of Nutrition & Foodservice Professionals and looks for ways to create jobs for association members.

III

Joyce Gilbert, PhD, RDN

President and CEO, Association of Nutrition & Foodservice Professionals

In 2013, Joyce Gilbert joined the now 15,000-member Association of Nutrition & Foodservice Professionals (ANFP) as president and chief executive officer. Almost 70% of ANFP members work in hospitals, long-term care, and senior dining. The vast majority are certified dietary managers, certified food protection professionals (CDM, CFPP).

Among the many hats Gilbert wears as the association's

chief staff leader is that of data strategist. "Big Data and AI [artificial intelligence] are the future," Gilbert notes. Data drive what ANFP communicates to its members, which helps the ANFP benchmark its long-term and acute-care practices with government guidelines and identify best practices.

"Technology—namely, continually gathering and mining data—is fueling our growth and future," Gilbert says. "It's important for our members to have access to and understand the value of Big Data and AI. But technology can be a struggle for some people, so we try to remove the complexity. Collaboration with other organizations, such as the Academy of Nutrition and Dietetics, is also important for collecting data, making it useful, and creating best practices. In other words, making [data] real to everyone."

―――

"Technology—namely, continually gathering and mining data—is fueling our growth and future."

―――

As Gilbert observes, "There are opportunities to make a difference in people's lives." The artful application of Big Data and AI is one of them.

I∥I

As a data-driven profession, the concept of Big Data is familiar to us. We rely on data in research, for outcomes information, and for designing communications and education strategies. Since 2014, the Academy of Nutrition and Dietetics Health Informatics Infrastructure (ANDHII) has offered dietitians tools to input, track, and report patient outcomes.[20] Through informatics—collecting and sharing clinical data—we can move the nutrition and dietetics profession forward, expand our opportunities, improve patient outcomes, and increase reimbursement funding for nutrition as a tool to prevent and manage disease. Using these data to help solve problems related to food waste and sustainability can also demonstrate the value of what we do in the community. This is just the beginning of how technology will influence our ability to document our value. It enables us to capture data from all areas of practice.

What Is Informatics?

Health informatics is a specialized field within health care that combines communications, technology, information, and health care with the goal of improving the care delivered to patients. Informatics uses health information systems to collect, store, retrieve, analyze, and apply information for common purposes, such as collaboration and coordination among providers.

The field of health informatics includes medical, nursing, pharmacy, dental, and public health. In today's rapidly changing environment, success in dietetics practice requires skill finding, evaluating, and sharing accurate food and nutrition information. In response, food and nutrition professionals are building nutrition informatics as a new area of dietetics practice.

Nutrition informatics manages nutrition data in combination with standards, processes, and technology to improve knowledge and practice, which in turn leads to improved quality of care and work efficiency.[21]

Artificial Intelligence

Artificial intelligence (AI) is discussed frequently when talking about the future of technology. If you have a voice-controlled virtual digital assistant such as Alexa or Siri in your home or business, you are already using artificial intelligence.

The term *artificial intelligence* was coined in 1956 at a Dartmouth College summer research project where scientists gathered to explore ways to make machines more "knowing" and to create a framework to better understand human intelligence, such as learning and problem solving. At the root of AI is the concept that the process of human thought can be mechanized.[21] AI is used to create efficiencies, boost productivity, and document outcomes. Data provide the fuel to implement AI.

In health care, including nutrition care, AI is used to analyze clinical data and combinations of data for disease diagnosis, progression, and treatment as well as for patient monitoring, outcomes research, and disease modeling. Personal digital health-management platforms, such as nutrition-related smart phone apps and wearable devices, generate data on patient activity and patient-reported outcomes. By integrating this information with preexisting data sets, AI can suggest treatment priorities according to real-time needs, produce intervention alerts, and recommend follow-up actions. As dietitians, these data will provide vast resources for us to apply in new and creative ways in varied settings.

AI is quickly having a profound influence on our profession. It will determine skills and education we need to integrate into our practice. Keeping abreast of new developments and how our employers plan to use AI now and in the future is essential. The ability of software to mimic how human brains work, particularly in developing neural networks, will play a big part in our field's future. A recent article in *The Wall Street Journal* gave examples of an electronic tongue with sensors that could identify the taste of a beverage and how machine learning can predict reactions to certain odors.[22] These certainly have implications for the food and beverage industry, but there are also applications in clinical situations to diagnose and manage disease, monitor patient response to treatment, and promote wellness in ways that are both more accurate and cost effective. Sensors and cameras on toilets that can look for disease can provide valuable information for public health, as well. We need to be aware of these innovations so we can be at the table guiding developments in yet another exciting pathway for a nutrition authority.

PERSONALIZED NUTRITION

Nutrition is often described as one of the most complex aspects of health care. As we learn more about individual differences and responses to therapies and interventions, some of our traditional recommendations may be challenged. Although medical professionals recognize that each patient is unique in terms of variables such as age, race, ethnicity, weight, and family history, they typically use diagnostic and treatment methods tailored to broad populations rather than individual patients. Advances in medicine and technology, however, are making precision medicine increasingly possible in treating patients with cancer, diabetes, cardiovascular disease, and other complex conditions. Precision nutrition is an area where we are needed to help interpret data and develop individual food and nutrition solutions.

Obesity is a condition that Jim Hill, PhD, thinks can benefit from precision nutrition. Hill thinks of obesity as the most prevalent health care problem in the country, if not the world. It is complex and requires a personalized approach that RDNs are in the best position to provide.

Like medical science, nutrition science has been based on the notion that everyone absorbs and metabolizes nutrients in similar ways, and that differences in daily requirements are mainly based on age, gender, and activity level. Now, however, we are learning more about variables such as lifestyle, gut microbiome, medications, and environment having a unique effect on each person's response to food and nutrients.

I | I

James O. Hill, PhD

Director, UAB Nutrition Obesity Research Center; Professor/Chairman, Department of Nutrition Sciences, School of Health Professions, University of Alabama at Birmingham

"This is a great time to be a dietitian," Jim Hill, director of the University of Alabama at Birmingham Nutrition Obesity Research Center, proclaims. "The research going on now, especially through the National Institutes of Health's Nutrition

122

for Precision within the 'All of Us' program, is going to yield so much data to help personalize nutrition counseling. Through the application of artificial intelligence to Big Data, registered dietitian nutritionists (RDNs) can assume a leadership position in determining what diet will be best for an individual."

"RDNs are the foot soldiers who can provide guidance as they customize instruction to their clients based on data uniquely suited to what may be referred to as 'precision nutrition."

"The barriers to solving the obesity problem have not been overcome in more than 30 years of trying. After claims made by one miracle diet after the next, we now recognize that many factors including exercise and behavior affect obesity. No one diet is right for everyone. RDNs are the foot soldiers who can provide guidance as they customize instruction to their clients based on data uniquely suited to what may be referred to as 'precision nutrition.' While dietitians need not understand every detail of the emerging research, they do need to appreciate the value these incredible tools bring to their work to help improve the health of the public. It's an exciting opportunity."

THE ROLE OF GENETICS IN PERSONALIZED NUTRITION

Under the umbrella of nutritional genomics, professionals in the fields of nutrigenomics and nutrigenetics study the relationship between diet and genes. Nutrigenetics is an aspect of personalized nutrition that studies different responses—such as weight, blood pressure, plasma cholesterol, and glucose levels—to a specific type of diet, depending on the individual's genotype. In contrast, nutrigenomics studies the interactions between diet and the expression of specific genes that keep the body healthy.[23]

"Nutritional genomics can be expected to revolutionize the way dietitians and other health professionals identify people with chronic diseases and treat those diseases," Milly Ryan-Harshman, PhD, writes. "Understanding the science of nutritional genomics is important to dietitians and other health professionals because major scientific advancements such as this usually have a significant impact on ethics, policy, and practice."[24]

According to Ruth DeBusk, PhD, RDN, and Yael Joffe, PhD, RD, FACN, authors of *It's Not Just Your Genes*, "We have the power to use the information encoded in our genes to help us make informed choices that will maximize our genetic potential.… Nutrition scientists, health care professionals, and every one of us has a stake in the continuing development of this field, based on our common desire to translate genetic information into practical prescriptions for personalized health care."[25]

Nutrition research continues to reveal the body's complex responses to individual nutrients and their interactions, and consumers increasingly demand answers to their nutrition and health questions. Food and nutrition professionals must be ready to bridge the gap by communicating to patients and clients what we are learning and by offering recommendations to help them. Consumers are reading all sorts of information online and via social media platforms; some is accurate, and some is not. We should be prepared to offer guidance on the best course of action that is currently known.

As Mary Rozga, PhD, RDN, and her colleagues Marie Latulippe, MS, RDN, and Alison Steiber, PhD, RDN, explain in "Advancements in Personalized Nutrition Technologies: Guiding Principles for Registered Dietitian Nutritionists," RDNs regularly practice a traditional type of personalized nutrition when they use the profession's nutrition care process to assess clients, either clinically or preventively, and collaborate with them to improve nutrition behaviors according to their needs and values, practitioner experience, and the best available evidence. In acute clinical settings, food and nutrition professionals use medical nutrition therapy (MNT)—often enteral and parenteral feeding—to treat patients with single or a combination of morbidities.[26]

Today, personalized nutrition assessment yields far more information than a standard blood panel, including behavioral and psychological data; genetic data; and microbiome, proteome, and metabolome data. Modeling technology can transform this information into personalized recommendations for diet and physical activity.

The National Institutes of Health (NIH) is the major funder of biomedical research in the United States. Its funding priorities reflect which health issues are considered major concerns. In 2016, NIH established the Nutrition Research Task Force to coordinate and accelerate nutrition research.[27] In 2020, the task force developed a strategic plan to advance nutrition research. One of the plan's objectives is to enable health care providers to recommend what, when, why, and how individuals should eat to optimize their health—an approach known as "precision nutrition."[28]

In this plan, Francis S. Collins, MD, PhD, former director of the NIH, explains[28]:

> *The nutrition research field is poised to make a leap forward by taking advantage of a lot of insights and technologies and rethinking the approach to answering those age-old questions about how food influences our health and what we can do about it.*

The task force plans to answer four major questions[28]:

1. What do we eat and how does it affect us?
2. What and when should we eat?
3. How does what we eat promote health across our lifespan?
4. How can we improve the use of food as medicine?

In line with the NIH, the Academy of Nutrition and Dietetics has developed a set of research priorities for the next decade. Priorities include nutrition-related discovery, clinical nutrition research, implementation, and public health.[29]

Big Data, artificial intelligence, and personal nutrition are changing the roles of nutrition and dietetics professionals. Global governments, public health organizations, private industry, and others are exploring how information technology impacts their business model, and so should we. For example, how we function in the future food system will be based on technologies that guide food production, distribution, and marketing. It is an exciting time to be in our profession. It is a time to open new doors for the profession and be receptive to new ways of doing our jobs. These changes require more of us—greater depth of knowledge, collaboration, and analytical skills and strong advocacy. High standards and attention to detail are among the hallmarks of our profession. These traits are valuable assets that have always underpinned our authority and credibility in times of rapid change.

The Academy of Nutrition and Dietetics has excellent resources for learning how to apply technology in various practice settings. Understanding the application of information technology in your own work setting and consulting with those who have expertise and insight are important steps toward recognizing and seizing opportunities along the new frontier of the nutrition and dietetics profession.

RESEARCH: THE FOUNDATION FOR THE FUTURE

Any discussion of the future of nutrition and dietetics needs to acknowledge the fundamental role research plays in the profession. Research has formed the backbone of dietetics practice and continues to serve as the foundation for the Academy of Nutrition and Dietetics work in professional and consumer education, advocacy, policy making, and strategic collaboration in the public and private sectors. Research in nutrition and dietetics improves patient care and outcomes by collecting, evaluating, and analyzing data from different interventions, thus providing a foundation for evidence-based practice. In their article on integrating nutrition science into basic and clinical research and care, Daniel J. Raiten, MD, Gerald F. Combs, PhD, Alison L. Steiber, PhD, RDN, and Andrew A. Bremer, MD, PhD, provide a valuable perspective on the evolution of the field of nutrition in an increasingly complex global health context where nutritional status is viewed as a biological variable.[30] Nutrition science, like all science, continues to evolve, and thus will always provide opportunities for RDNs to explore new frontiers in the profession.

Some nutrition and dietetics professionals use study results to craft messages and give advice to patients; others work as researchers behind the scenes, providing the evidence base that underpins informed practice. No matter where you are engaged in practice, it is our shared responsibility to keep current on science and participate in demonstrating and expanding our knowledge and value. Recognizing the role of applied research in our profession is essential to our being trusted as professionals and recognized as authorities. The Academy of Nutrition and Dietetics 2020 Research Priorities Report reminds us of the myriad ways research improves patient care.[29]

As you participate in professional meetings and webinars and read the literature, you get a glimpse into emerging topics that will affect all of us as professionals. You probably have a list of topics that interest you. You and your RDN colleagues have the opportunity to contribute to growing bodies of evidence in diverse areas within the field.

One area where interest is high is the gut microbiome. The influence of diet on gut health is a complex area. What works well for one individual may have little or no impact on another. For example, if you have counseled patients who have received a diagnosis of irritable bowel syndrome, you are aware that recommendations such as increasing fiber and prebiotics/probiotics in the diet works for some individuals, but not all. In situations like this, personal or precision nutrition comes into play. Variables such as food types, dietary patterns, behavior, health status, and so on, all contribute to the big picture.

Because food is our therapeutic tool, we must know, in some detail, what is in it. Although many databases are available, we require more detailed information on food composition, including, for example, phytochemicals and metabolites. In addition, databases must be integrated to help researchers achieve greater clarity on the effects of diet. Artificial intelligence has facilitated linkages and integration among databases. Private industry is a key partner in providing product information. Emerging technology will offer new methods of testing and organizing food data, all of which can transform nutrition research and provide significant evidence for diet intervention in areas like the gut.

The brain is another increasingly important area of study about which consumers have questions. The gut microbiome produces hormones and neurotransmitters, which are messengers to the brain that regulate the emotions and stresses of daily living. The emerging field of nutritional psychiatry looks at the role diet and the gut microbiome play in shaping mood, mental illness, and depression.

The preponderance of research related to the brain is on dementia or Alzheimer disease (AD). As the population ages, AD is the sixth leading cause of death in the United States, a major cost to the health care system, and a heartbreak to families.[31]

In a 2021 *Forbes* interview, Martha M. Boudreau, COO at the 38-million-member AARP, notes that people aged 85 years and older comprise the fastest-growing population segment; the second fastest is people aged 100 years and over.[32] If you are 50 years old and in good health, half of your life (statistically speaking) is ahead of you. These numbers drive home the value of starting disease prevention early with diet and of conducting more research in this area; they also illustrate the growing opportunities for nutrition professionals now and in the future in gerontologic and long-term care research on diseases that impact people aged 65 and over (such as diseases of the heart and lungs, and diabetes).

Researchers are investigating highly processed foods; foods high in sugar, refined carbohydrates, and unhealthy fat; as well as the presence of phytochemicals that mitigate age-related oxidative stress. In addition, trials are looking at the connection between DHA (omega-3 fatty acids) and amyloid deposits in the brain. Some of this research may reveal dietary changes that influence efforts to prevent disease. For example, Mediterranean diets cause less brain pathology in people with AD than do diets high in saturated fat.[33] The Mediterranean diet, the Nordic diet, and other plant-based diets rich in foods like fish, whole grains, nuts, and olive oil and low in refined carbohydrates and sugar offer promise. The message is that nutrition research is complex, involving many biological factors.

The research issues highlighted here are examples of many that reveal opportunities for nutrition and dietetics professionals to engage in research or help translate the best science into practice. Research is a link to our future in all career paths and areas of practice. Now is the time to demonstrate the value of RDNs in many aspects of science. The NIH's engagement in nutrition research as reflected in its strategic plan and increasing interest in the latest nutrition research in the global marketplace provide a platform for demonstrating our authority.[34]

REFERENCES

1. Chronic conditions. Centers for Medicare & Medicaid Services website. Accessed October 21, 2021. www.cms.gov/Research-Statistics-Data-and -Systems/Statistics-Trends-and-Reports/Chronic-Conditions/CC_Main
2. About chronic diseases. National Health Council website. Accessed October 21, 2021. https://nationalhealthcouncil.org/wp-content/uploads/2019/12 /AboutChronicDisease.pdf
3. About chronic diseases. Centers for Disease Control and Prevention. Accessed October 21, 2021. www.cdc.gov/chronicdisease/about/index.htm
4. Hunger in America. Feeding America website. Accessed October 21, 2021. www.feedingamerica.org/hunger-in-america
5. The Nutrition Impact Summit. Academy of Nutrition and Dietetics Foundation website. Accessed October 25, 2021. www.eatrightfoundation.org /why-it-matters/second-century/nutrition-impact-summit

6. *Nutrition and Food Systems.* The High Level Panel of Experts on Food Security and Nutrition of the Committee on World Food Security; 2017. Accessed December 20, 2020. www.fao.org/fileadmin/user_upload/hlpe/hlpe _documents/HLPE_Reports/HLPE-Report-12_EN.pdf

7. The 17 goals. United Nations Department of Economic and Social Affairs, Sustainable Development. 2015. Accessed December 20, 2020. https://sdgs .un.org/goals

8. What is sustainability? UCLA Sustainability website. 2020. Accessed December 20, 2020. www.sustain.ucla.edu/what-is-sustainability

9. United Nations. Decade of Action on Nutrition (2016-2025) website. Accessed December 20, 2020. www.un.org/nutrition

10. Spiker M, Knoblock-Hahn A. Cultivating sustainable, resilient, and healthy food and water systems: A nutrition-focused framework for action. *J Acad Nutr Diet.* 2020;120(6):1057-1067.

11. Blankenship J, Smith Brown R. Food system sustainability: An Academy advocacy priority. *J Acad Nutr Diet.* 2020; 120(6):1054-1056.

12. Branca F, Demaio A, Udomkesmalee E, et al. A new nutrition manifesto for a new nutrition reality. *Lancet.* 2020;395(10217):8-10. doi:10.1016/S0140 -6736(19)32690-X

13. One third of poorer countries face both undernutrition and obesity: WHO report. World Health Organization. December 16, 2019. Accessed May 6, 2022. https://news.un.org/en/story/2019/12/1053571?msclkid=045d70 fec4db11ecbc6a5bd6e3fc6fc0

14. Vogliano C, Steiber A, Brown K. Linking agriculture, nutrition, and health: The role of the Registered Dietitian Nutritionist. *J Acad Nutr Diet.* 2015;115(10):1710-1714.

15. International Food Information Council. 2020 Food and Health Survey. Food Insight website. 2019. Accessed December 20, 2020. https://foodinsight.org /wp-content/uploads/2020/06/IFIC-Food-and-Health-Survey-2020.pdf

16. Office for the Advancement of Telehealth. Health Resources & Services Administration website. Accessed July 20, 2021. www.hrsa.gov/rural-health /telehealth

17. Academy unveils telehealth stance for use in policy and advocacy initiatives. Academy of Nutrition and Dietetics website. April 12, 2021. Accessed October 25, 2021. https://www.eatrightpro.org/news-center/on-the-pulse-of-public -policy/from-the-hill/academy-unveils-telehealth-stance-for-use-in-policy -and-advocacy-initiatives

18. Rose S, Hurwitz HM, Mercer MB, et al. Patient experience in virtual visits hinges on technology and the patient-clinician relationship: A large survey study with open-ended questions. *J Med Internet Res.* 2021;23(6):e18488. doi:10.2196/18488

19. Jain A. The five Vs of Big Data. IBM website. Accessed November 6, 2021. www.ibm.com/blogs/watson-health/the-5-vs-of-big-data

20. Position of the Academy of Nutrition and Dietetics: Nutrition informatics. *J Acad Nutr Diet.* 2019;119(8):1375-1382.

21. Smith C, McGuire B, Huang T, Yang G. The history of artificial intelligence. University of Washington Computer Science & Engineering course website. December 2006. Accessed December 20, 2020. https://courses.cs.washington .edu/courses/csep590/06au/projects/history-ai.pdf

22. Loren A, Hand K. How computers with humanlike senses will change our lives. The Wall Street Journal website. July 9, 2021. Accessed April 25, 2022. www.wsj.com/articles/how-computers-with-humanlike-senses-will-change-our -lives-11625760066

23. Mutch DM, Wahli W, Williamson G. Nutrigenomics and nutrigenetics: the emerging faces of nutrition. *FASEB J.* 2005;19(12):1602-16. doi:10.1096/fj .05-3911rev

24. Ryan-Harshman M, Vogel E, Jones-Taggart H, et al. Nutritional genomics and dietetic professional practice. *Can J Diet Pract Res.* 2008;69(4):177-182.

25. DeBusk R, Joffe, Y. *It's Not Just Your Genes.* BKDR, Inc; 2006.

26. Rozga M, Latulippe M, Steiber A. Advancements in personalized nutrition technologies: Guiding principles for registered dietitian nutritionists. *J Acad Nutr Diet.* 2020;120(6):1074-1085.

27. NIH task force formed to develop first nutrition strategic plan. News release. National Institutes of Health. October 1, 2016. Accessed October 21, 2021. www.nih.gov/news-events/news-releases/nih-task-force-formed-develop-first -nutrition-strategic-plan

28. Viguers S. New NIH research goals focus on "precision nutrition." Healio website. 2020. Accessed December 20, 2020. www.healio.com/news/primary -care/20200602/new-nih-research-goals-focus-on-precision-nutrition

29. Academy of Nutrition and Dietetics. *Academy Research Priorities: An Agenda to Advance Nutrition and Dietetics Knowledge and Practice.* eatrightPRO website. 2020. Accessed December 20, 2020. www.eatrightpro.org/-/media/eatrightpro -files/research/research-priorities-final-report.pdf

30. Raiten D, Combs GF, Steiber AL, Bremer AA. Perspective: Nutritional status as a biological variable (NABV): Integrating nutrition science into basic and clinical research and care. *Adv Nutr.* 2021;12(5):1599-1609. doi:10.1093 /advances/nmab046

31. Alzheimer's disease facts and figures. Alzheimer's Association website. Accessed October 30, 2021. www.alz.org/media/Documents/alzheimers-facts-and -figures.pdf

32. Knox D. How AARP guided their members through the pandemic. *Forbes*. April 27, 2021. Accessed April 25, 2022. www.forbes.com/sites/daveknox /2021/04/27/how-aarp-guided-their-members-through-the-pandemic /?sh=1a8a4f23dd51

33. Ballarini T, Melo van Lent D, Brunner J, et al. Mediterranean diet, Alzheimer disease biomarkers, and brain atrophy in old age. *Neurology*. June 15, 2021;9(54).

34. *2020-2030 Strategic plan for NIH nutrition research*. National Institute of Health Office of Nutrition Research; 2020. Accessed December 20, 2020. https://dpcpsi.nih.gov/onr/strategic-plan

III

Epilogue

Writing *Nutrition Authority: Perspectives on Opportunity* allowed me to share my thoughts on what makes an authority in nutrition and dietetics. Interviews with successful registered dietitian nutritionists and outside experts and insights gleaned from the literature and scientific publications further illuminated what it takes to be a trusted authority. While there are many aspects to nutrition authority, I highlighted only a few of the points I believe to be important.

I hope this book accomplishes two goals: to stimulate discussions among you and your colleagues and organizations about what is necessary to be a trusted authority, and to assist you in identifying ways to help the profession remain a respected authority in food and nutrition in this environment of challenge and change.

Knowledge, Communication, and Collaboration: Essential Elements

No doubt all of us agree: knowledge, especially in one's area of practice, is a major requirement for success in our profession. The Academy of Nutrition and Dietetics Center for Lifelong Learning, annual Food & Nutrition Conference & Expo (FNCE) conference, and dietetic practice groups offer opportunities to strengthen our professional expertise and knowledge base. Specialist certifications and the shift to establishing a master's degree as the base of entry into the profession underscore the importance of deepening our knowledge and the need to be aware of the latest scientific research shaping food and nutrition practice.

Being aware of what is communicated in social media helps us identify areas where we should understand the dialogue and popular points of view. This is where discussions with colleagues from varied backgrounds can help form your perspective; where reading research broadly can help further understanding in major areas of interest; and where making referrals to registered dietitian nutritionists (RDNs) who have the needed expertise makes sense.

Being an authority also requires us to communicate knowledge in an empathic, effective, and convincing manner. Whether in a planned presentation or one-on-one counseling with a patient, begin with what you want the person or group to remember or base their action on. There may be many unanswered questions and differing views or recommended actions. Many of those interviewed here urge us to enter conversations, share our viewpoints, and refuse to shy away from conflict. People need to hear our views on science, which reinforce our authority.

The need for collaboration is a critical point made by those I interviewed. Having read the interviews, you were exposed to diverse perspectives that may help you shape your position as a nutrition authority. In my career, collaboration was essential. Joining forces with others and having them confirm your expertise is a credible way to position yourself as an authority. I can think of many examples where collaboration has been pivotal; for example, an RDN who engaged with the medical staff regarding the need for dietitian involvement on a clinical team; a community program that was marketed to other agencies to engage clients through joint programming; and a well-respected health care organization agreeing to assist in securing reimbursement for nutrition services. Having others speak on our behalf is fundamental to our ability to be included at the table and to enter new markets.

HISTORY, SCIENCE, AND NEW FRONTIERS: MY HOPES FOR THE PROFESSION

My goal in writing this book was to share my perspective on what it takes to be a nutrition authority. This is a broad topic, so I selected three areas or themes to guide my writing—history, science, and new frontiers of the future. The messages of those I interviewed are integrated into this platform.

Now that you have read *Nutrition Authority: Perspectives on Opportunity,* I hope you can see the connections between the history of the profession and the many forces that shaped who RDNs are today. What came before has application to how we move into the future. Mark Twain is credited with saying history doesn't often repeat itself, but it rhymes.[1] The qualities and actions that propelled us forward over the past centuries are still needed today: bold action, vision, challenging the system, and leveraging the moment are as relevant today as they were at our beginning. We must move to take advantage when windows of opportunity are open. They are not open forever; change happens fast.

I also hope this book has reinforced the fact that science—a process of discovery and change—underpins our profession. Keeping current, knowing what to communicate and how, is important to all RDNs, regardless of area of practice. The voice of the RDN must be heard.

Lastly, I hope that you will see how your interests and responsibilities fit into a big picture. While all of us have many interests and areas of expertise and practice, there is a critical need to see the whole landscape if we are to be major players as nutrition authorities. Since food and nutrition therapy are our tools, looking at where you fit in the food system may help you see how interdependent we are.

Writing about the future is a daunting task. Changes in how food is grown, produced, and marketed are driven by technologic advances in the food system. Technology also influences how information is used and how health care is provided now and moving forward. Technology offers a future in which we can prosper.

I wish you all success on the paths you take moving forward. The role of the nutrition professional has never been more important. Your success determines the future of the profession and that of the Academy of Nutrition and Dietetics. My hope is that forthcoming generations in our profession will build on the innovations and value you create as nutrition authorities today.

REFERENCE

1.   Sommer J. Funny, but I've heard this market song before. *New York Times*. June 11, 2011.

III

Continuing Professional Education

This edition of *Nutrition Authority: Perspectives on Opportunity* offers readers 2.5 hours of Continuing Professional Education (CPE) credit. Readers may earn credit by completing the interactive quiz at:

https://publications.webauthor.com/nutritionauthority